TIPS FOR EFFECTIVE COMMUNICATION

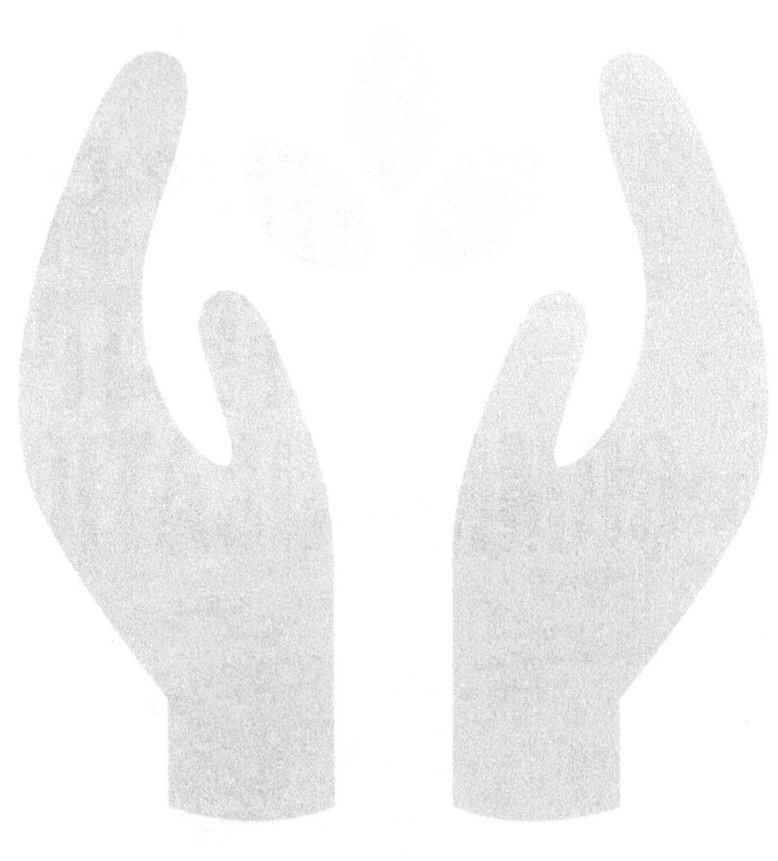

TIPS FOR EFFECTIVE COMMUNICATION

A VITAL TOOL FOR TRUST DEVELOPMENT IN HEALTHCARE

NONYE TOCHI AGHANYA

MSC, RN, FNP-C

TIPS FOR EFFECTIVE COMMUNICATION: A VITAL TOOL FOR TRUST DEVELOPMENT IN HEALTHCARE
Copyright © 2021 Nonye Tochi Aghanya, MSc, RN, FNP-C

All rights reserved. No part of this book may be used or reproduced by any means, graphic, electronic, or mechanical, including photocopying, recording, taping or by any information storage retrieval system without the written permission of the author except in the case of brief quotations embodied in critical articles and reviews.
Because of the dynamic nature of the Internet, any web addresses or links contained in this book may have changed since publication and may no longer be valid. The views expressed in this work are solely those of the author and do not necessarily reflect the views of the publisher, and the publisher hereby disclaims any responsibility for them.

ISBN: 9798727375693
Imprint: Independently published

Independent author published date: 04/01/2021

The information, ideas, and suggestions in this book are not intended as a substitute for professional advice. Before following any suggestions contained in this book, consult your physician or mental-health professional. Neither the author nor the publisher shall be liable or responsible for any loss or damage allegedly arising as a consequence of your use or application of any information or suggestions in this book.

Although these are real patient encounters, please note that scenarios, names, and locations are disguised to maintain privacy. No association with any actual patient is intended or should be inferred.

BUT THERE IS A SPIRIT IN MAN: AND THE INSPIRATION OF THE ALMIGHTY GIVETH THEM UNDERSTANDING.

JOB 32:8

TO MY FOUR DAUGHTERS, FROM WHOM
I'VE LEARNED THE LIFE SKILLS FOR
DAILY LIVING. THANK YOU.

CHICHI: MY DEFIANCE
YABA: MY STRENGTH
DIANE: MY COMPASSION
SARAH: MY PERSISTENCE

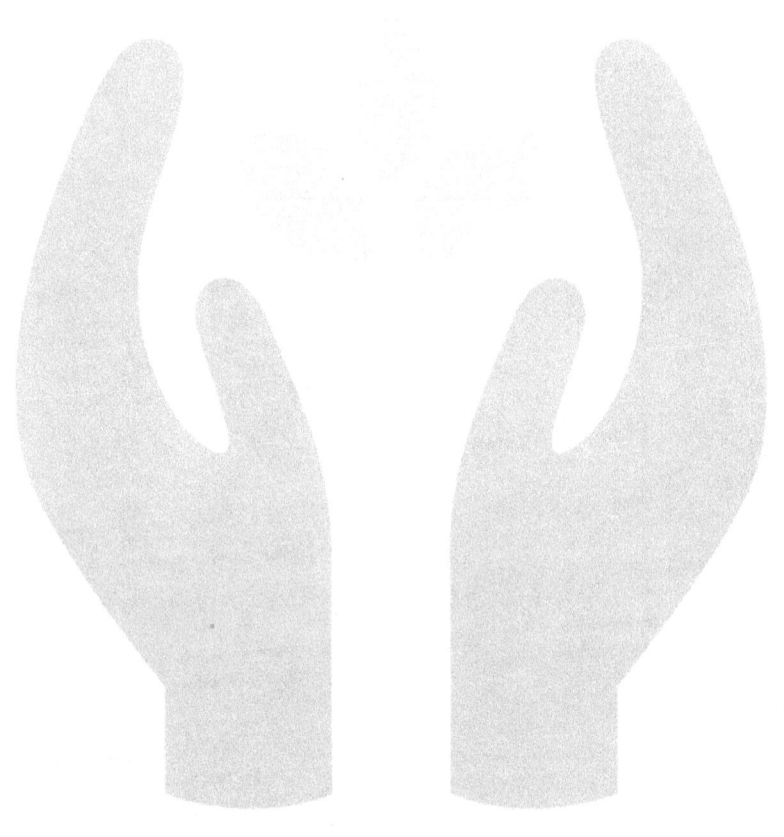

CONTENTS

CONTENTS IX
INTRODUCTION 1
CHAPTER ONE 7
For the Patient 7
   Simple Tips to Promote a Pleasant Clinic Visit with Your Clinician 9
   Dos 9
   Don'ts 11
      CHAPTER TWO 15
For Clinicians and Future Clinicians 15
      CHAPTER THREE 19
Talk to me, Doctor 19
Cognitive Memory 23
Emotional Memory 23
Patient Adherence 25
Clinician-Patient Positioning 27
Use of Patient Information 29
      CHAPTER FOUR 33
Hello, Patient ... but Who Are You? 33
      CHAPTER FIVE 39
The AngryPatient 39
      CHAPTER SIX 45
   The Opinionated (Overly Confident)Patient 45
      CHAPTER SEVEN 55
The DependentPatient 55
      CHAPTER EIGHT 61
The SkepticalPatient 61
      CHAPTER NINE 67

The SuspiciousPatient 67

CHAPTER TEN 71
The TalkativePatient 71

CHAPTER ELEVEN 77
The Dr. Moms and Dr. Dads 77

Common Don'ts 85

Rather, Practice These Common Dos 85

CHAPTER TWELVE 87
The Overwhelmed Patient 87

CHAPTER THIRTEEN 91
The ImpatientPatient 91

CHAPTER FOURTEEN 95
WhenthePatientIsa Health Care Provider 95

CHAPTER FIFTEEN 99
Communicating News of Terminal Illness to a Patient 99

CHAPTER SIXTEEN 103
The Adolescent Patient 103

CHAPTER SEVENTEEN 107
The Medical Patient with a Mental-Health Challenge 107

CHAPTER EIGHTEEN 113
DiscussingWeightwith the ObesePatient 113

CHAPTER NINETEEN 119
The Electronically Savvy Patient 119

Do You Know You Can Do More with Your Electronic Devices? 120

CHAPTER TWENTY 125
The Defiant Patient (the Aging Parent) 125

CHAPTER TWENTY-ONE 131
The "Normal"Patient 131

CHAPTER TWENTY-TWO 133
Review of Empirical Studies 133

Abstract 133

Introduction	134
The Problem	136
Method & Significance of Study	136
Literature Review	137
Review of Empirical Studies	140
REFERENCES	145

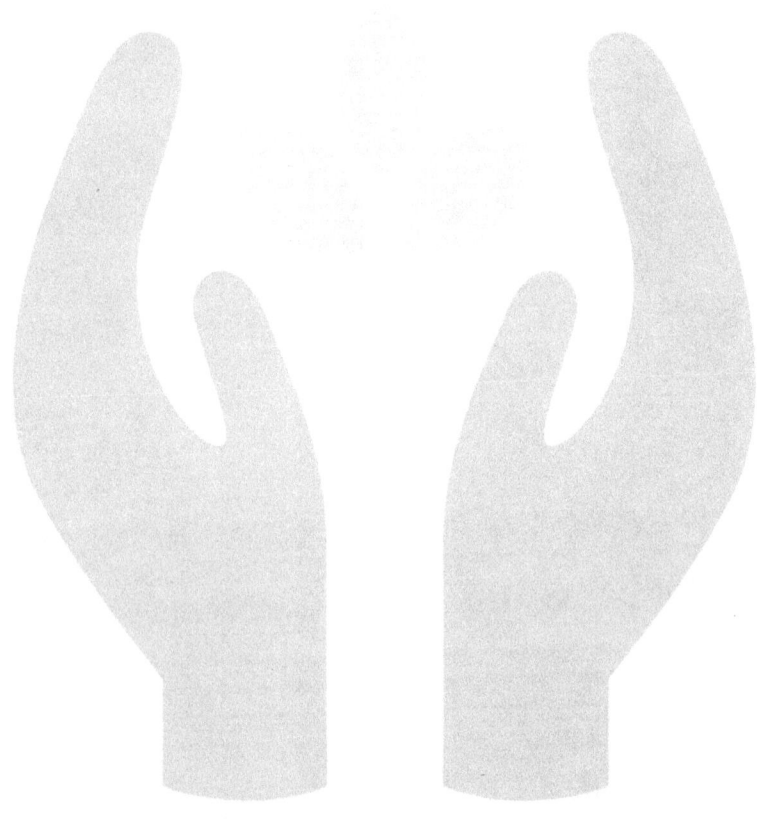

XII

INTRODUCTION

Please permit me to say that I procrastinated for a while about writing a book. When I finally decided to write a book (by the way, this is my first one ever—yeah!), I did some research to see whether any other book in circulation explored clinician-patient communication and that relationship. This is a very important topic, so there had to be, right?

If you guessed yes, you are right because I came across several books. This made me wonder whether I should even bother writing another to add to the circulation. However, as I further researched the other books, I did not come across any books with direct insight on this important topic from my perspective. My perspective is one of a practicing clinician who, as a recent patient, had the experience of interacting with various medical staff and other clinicians in several specialties during my period of recovery from a major surgical procedure. As a practicing clinician, I have interacted with many patients with different traits and personalities in diverse health care settings. Despite the attempts of many books to explore and identify factors and barriers that influence communication between patients and clinicians, many patients still do not feel comfortable talking freely to their clinicians. Thus, they find it difficult to have honest, open communication with their clinicians. In a recent online article at *Live Science*, statistics show that America's trust in the medical profession has decreased in recent years, well below other countries' public attitudes toward doctors. In a polled survey in 2012, fewer people said that they had great confidence in the leaders of the medical profession (only 34 percent of adults) than in 1996 (76 percent). Also, reports of a similar survey of people across twenty-nine countries show that the United States ranked twenty-fourth in public trust of doctors, well below Switzerland and Denmark (Harding 2014).

When I reviewed these results, I said to myself, "Wow, this is such a staggering number of unsatisfied patients." To the best of my knowledge, most (if not all) clinicians strive to maintain a decent and acceptable level of professionalism during clinician-patient consultations. So what could be the problem? Why such a staggering number of dissatisfied patients?

The reality is that the common communication style of most clinicians, although polite, pleasant, professional, and nonthreatening, has been insufficient in improving current statistics. Regardless of how nonthreatening a clinician's approach is, many patients still view the clinician as an authoritative figure, and thus they are more likely to feel intimidated by the clinician's presence. This can become a contributory factor to the patient's reservations during consultation visits. It means that more information needs to be made available to assist clinicians in developing specific communication skills that are applicable to the various patients they encounter each day in the health care system.

With funny illustrations of clinician-patient scenarios and simple dialogues, this guidebook highlights several patient personalities and the effects of those personalities as either strengths or barriers to forming a meaningful clinician-patient relationship. It provides the clinician with the needed communication tools to connect with all patients regardless of a patient's personality. This is the key to having an honest communication that results in a productive clinician-patient relationship. Clinicians must refrain from using a one-size-fits-all communication approach because patients have different personalities, and they typically perceive and react to the same information differently. For effective communication to be accomplished, the communication style must be tailored to each patient's personality.

Tips for Effective Communication: A Vital Tool for Trust Development

With patients' dwindling trust in their clinicians, it is fair to say that gone are the years when great manners, politeness, and professionalism were the only requirements a clinician needed to engage a patient in honest, open communication. This book also highlights and addresses several patient traits and personalities, as well as the effects of these personalities in promoting or deterring effective communication in health care settings. It is an informative tool that is a must-read for everyone (including patients, students in health department sectors, clinicians, and especially future clinicians). Not until we all truly understand one another's perspectives and contributions to the dynamics of clinician-patient relationships will a sincere and rewarding interaction be realized by both patients and clinicians. By applying the principle guidelines in this book, each party will be one step closer to achieving a fulfilling clinical experience.

So why did I finally decide to write a book? The answer is a simple one. I decided it was time to seriously address this problem, because in my thirty years of interacting with patients, I've noticed more patients ask me, "Can you please be my doctor?" Quite frankly, there needs to be a better form of communication between clinicians and patients in order for genuine trust to develop between both parties.

In 1990, when I graduated from the University of Nsukka, Nigeria, with a degree of Bachelor of Science in computer science, I did not imagine in my wildest dreams the role that computer informatics would play in meeting the ever-growing challenges of health care management. My BSc curriculum involved the study of such older programming languages as Basic, Fortran, Cobol, and Pascal. Following my arrival in the United States of America in 1991, I was not certain how I could apply my BSc in the workforce. I wasn't sure what to do with these old programming languages I had studied. In 1992, I abandoned my search for a profession in the computer informatics field and embarked on a journey to explore what contributions I could make in the health care field. Thirty years later, I am thankful that the world of computer science has further merged with health care management, resulting in an efficient mode of health care delivery through electronic health record systems.

I began my career as a nurse's assistant. Let's face it: a nurse's assistant interacts with a patient much differently than a clinician would. And in many instances, the average patient is not intimidated by a nurse's presence. Following my arrival to the United States, I soon worked as a nurse's assistant. However, there was one problem: I was terrified of interacting with the patients! I was constantly conscious of the fact that I needed to speak and act in a proper manner in order to make the patients feel comfortable around me. I remember that many patients were eager to assist me in feeling comfortable around them. Some asked me if I'd recently migrated to the United States, asked what language I spoke and wanted to learn about my country, Nigeria. There was a genuine curiosity and interest from the patients as they asked these questions.

It was at this moment that I came up with the phrase "true self" because I noticed that these patients whom I cared for while I performed my role as a nurse's assistant were always their true selves. They did not need to work hard to please me; rather, asking me questions to genuinely know me was an attempt on their part to help me become my true self and feel comfortable around them. They wanted to know who I was as a human being, rather than as someone who cared for them and assisted them with their activities of daily living. During those early years, I got my first opportunity to observe patient behaviors and engage with my patients in honest, heart-to-heart conversations about their lives, families, and future goals. Patient communication during this period was usually spontaneous, friendly, and stress-free and the interactions often benefited both the patients and me. If you get nothing else from this book, please don't miss this important fact: the goal of every clinician should be to assist the patient to come to a state of true self and aim to interact with patients when patients are their true selves. This is because patients are more honest, forthcoming, transparent, and compliant, and they ask questions when they are their true selves. This is the basis for a productive clinician-patient interaction.

After two years as a nurse's assistant, I realized that there had to be more I could do to help patients beyond my duties as a nurse's assistant. I became a licensed practical nurse and later went on to become a registered nurse. As a registered nurse, I was able to interact in more detail with my patients and was no longer limited to discussions about their pastime activities. I was now able to discuss their health progress and medications, I realized that I was becoming more of an authority figure to my patients than when I was a nurse's assistant, but the personal traits of compassion, warmth, kindness, patience, and empathy that I had cultivated during my years as a nurse's assistant were already embedded in me.

For the next eight years as a registered nurse, I encountered many patients and their families in the hospital, long-term care, subacute, and home-care settings. One particularly interesting thing I noticed was that patients would readily tell me their symptoms but were frequently hesitant to disclose the same information to their doctors. Although I would disclose these patients' reports to their doctors, the knowledge of this lapse in communication further inspired me to advance my education and become a clinician. It's because as a registered nurse, I wasn't at liberty to diagnose and provide medical treatment to these patients who were eager to disclose their symptoms to me but not to their doctors.

When I became a family nurse practitioner in 2001, I had finally come full circle in gaining a true understanding of patient traits and personalities and the impacts these traits can have in helping to establish a productive clinician-patient relationship—or in deterring the development of such a relationship. I can truly say that my various experiences have enabled me to acquire the skills of applying a specific interaction approach to assist the most difficult patient to feel comfortable in my presence. As an active family nurse practitioner, I look forward each day to meeting my patients because the knowledge and skills I've developed over thirty years also enable me to make each patient consultation a pleasant and rewarding one for both the patient and me. This led to the writing of this simple guidebook so that other clinicians may learn the strategic steps necessary to developing an effective, productive, and rewarding clinician-patient relationship.

I wish to thank all the patients that I've had the honor to have several encounters within various health care settings for the past thirty years. I am truly a more thoughtful and caring clinician, a caring wife and mother, and an overall better human being because of all of you. In a world where more people are silently hurting and in dire need of sincere, compassionate interactions, I thank my Lord and Savior; Jesus Christ and the Holy Spirit, for giving me the inspiration to write this book as my contribution in helping many people in need for compassionate care.

Finally, I thank my wonderful husband, JJ, for his patience and support through many nights that I suddenly awoke from deep sleep with ideas I just had to write down.

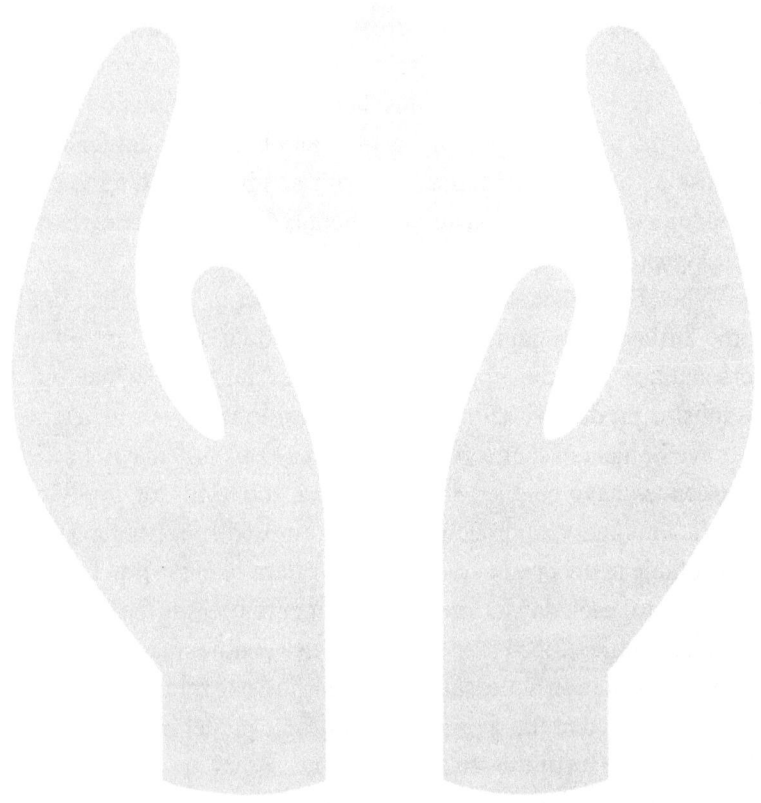

CHAPTER ONE

For the Patient

As you read this book, you may not be a patient at this moment in your life but chances are that you have probably visited with a clinician at some point in the past few years, or you may even have an upcoming scheduled clinician's appointment. In addition, you might know of a family member, friend, or coworker who has been a patient in the health care system. Let's face it: as grim as it sounds, the reality is that at some point in your life, you will need the assistance of a clinician to address an acute illness, maintain adequate management of a chronic illness, or get a general health physical examination.

Have you ever asked yourself, "Why does it seem as though my clinician never utterly understands me? Why do I feel like I cannot open up and have a heart-to-heart conversation with my clinician? Why do I feel terrified when I go to my clinician's office?" If you have, know that you are not alone. These are only a few of the many common concerns that we face as patients in the health care system. This book, in a simple, straightforward pattern, attempts to bring to light some of the factors that can either hinder or promote the development of a trusting, productive, and rewarding clinician-patient relationship. I encourage everyone to read this book in its entirety because information contained within each page reveals the dos and don'ts from both the patient's and the clinician's perspective, which can contribute to improving communication while promoting trust between both parties. I surely hope that patients will share this book with their clinicians and vice versa.

It is important for you as a patient to understand that although most clinicians strive to maintain a high level of professionalism during consultation visits, it is typically not the only factor that is required in order for you to feel a connection with the clinician. As a patient, what does it mean to feel that you connected with your clinician? At the end of a consultation visit, if you leave the clinician's office with more questions than answers, there was probably not much of a connection. In addition, if you feel you could not speak up, or that if you did speak and disclose your opinions but you were not heard, or that the visit was rushed—or heck, if you feel the clinician came in with her mind already made up about what your problem was, then you did not make a connection with that clinician. The information within this book provides tips to help patients achieve a more fulfilled visit with their clinicians. More importantly, it also gives some guidelines for clinicians to apply that will help them to understand different patients' perspectives.

As Forrest Gump said, "Life is like a box of chocolates: you never know what you are going to get." In life, unforeseen circumstances can suddenly change one's role from a clinician to a patient. When a medical care provider suddenly becomes a patient and seeks medical care in the health care field, a lot of psychological changes take place that can alter the existing perspectives of that medical care provider with regards to the general health care delivery system.

I know from firsthand experience what it feels like to wear a hat: both for a clinician and a patient. After many years of practicing as a family nurse practitioner and enjoying good health for most of my adult years, I suddenly discovered that I needed to have surgery for the repair of an abdominal hernia and the removal of an exceptionally large fibroid that had made it quite challenging for me to bend down without excruciating pain. In 2013, I underwent a major abdominal surgery and was unable to return to work for five months following the surgery. During this period of recovery, I traded my clinician hat for that of a patient. Although I believed I had always efficiently interacted with several of my patients through my professional years,

I sincerely felt for the first time what it really meant to be a patient. As an active mother of four girls, I was terrified of the unknown that is typically associated with surgical routines requiring general anesthesia. So many questions flooded my mind. "Will I still be okay when I wake up? Who will care for my family as I recover?" (Thanks to my loving husband, that issue was taken care of, but it still did not make me worry any less!)

Following the surgery, I realized that I was equally terrified of the recovery process, which involved follow-up tests, scans, doctor's appointments, and more. It was during this recovery process that it finally clicked for me. I concluded that as a patient, there is a train of thought process and expected behaviors that will promote the development of a productive and trusting relationship with clinicians. As a clinician, I have always known that I must abide by certain codes and ethics in order to provide optimal care to my patients. But it was not until I spent a great deal of time as a patient in the health care system that it dawned on me that a trusting relationship cannot be successfully achieved in a unilateral format by either the patient or the clinician. It is a joint venture and a two-way street. Both parties must be willing to hold each other to a higher standard of conduct and participate wholeheartedly in the process of developing a successful clinician-patient relationship. I am happy to say that with the help of my wonderful doctors, and surely by the grace of God, I made a successful recovery and am back to caring for my patients, but not before I learnt some valuable lessons that now help me better relate to my patients.

Simple Tips to Promote a Pleasant Clinic Visit with Your Clinician

Dos
- Strive to keep your scheduled clinic appointments.
- Maintain an optimistic attitude with the clinical experience.
- Take your list of current medications to your clinic appointments.

- Write down a list of questions you wish to ask the staff and the clinician.
- Inform your clinician of any medical changes since your last visit.
- Bring up concerns on topics you feel the clinician may have missed.

Although these may seem like very simple instructions, it is important to note that many mistakes can occur, and important points are missed when these instructions are not consistently implemented or are ignored. Keeping up with your scheduled appointments reassures the clinician that you are diligent about taking care of your health. It is a bit discouraging for the clinician to have a patient who repeatedly cancels scheduled appointments. These patients are sometimes referred to as frequent "no-shows". Occasional cancellation of an appointment is expected, but perpetual cancellation could be interpreted as nonchalance in contributing to the health plan.

Prior to your scheduled appointment, write down a list of questions and concerns that you wish to discuss during your clinic visit. The clinic environment can be an intimidating one for many people. Usually, prior to your consultation with the clinician, your initial contact could be with other clinic staff members that would ask questions pertaining to your visit. It is important to itemize your questions and provide the front desk staff with up-to-date responses to questions regarding insurance coverage.

Following my surgical procedure and during my period of recovery as a patient, I noticed that maintaining a friendly and welcoming attitude on arrival to clinic appointments helped ease some of my anxiety which led to easier interactions with all staff. It is important to note that polite and cheerful interactions with the front desk staff lifts your spirit and helps set the tone for the remainder of your clinical visit with other clinic staff members, including the clinician. Provide the nursing staff with information about any changes in medications, allergies, immunizations, discharge papers regarding recent hospitalizations, lab results, x-rays, and other scan reports.

Avoid distractions during the clinical consult with your clinician. If possible, turn off cell phones and other electronic devices. Keep an open mind as you talk to your clinician. In a straightforward manner, state your concerns, fears, and reservations concerning your medical complaints and treatment plans. Refer to your list of questions if you feel you missed any point of concern. If applicable, inform the clinician that updated medical lists were provided to the nursing staff so that all issues can be addressed. When you are not satisfied with a diagnosis or plan of medical care, remember that you have the right to seek a second opinion. Still, maintain an appreciative attitude for your clinician's efforts.

Follow up with your clinician's office to obtain results of recent tests performed during your visit, and to determine whether you need to set up follow-up appointments to discuss those results with your clinician.

Don'ts

- Do not get into the habit of self-diagnosis prior to a clinic visit.
- Do not be rude to the clinic staff.
- Do not distract the clinician.
- Do not rush the clinical visit.
- Don't be scared of the clinical visit experience.

It is unwise to perform extensive Internet research for minor ailments such as rash, cough, sore throat, and ear pain prior to your initial appointment with your clinician. You will learn of other differential diagnosis (other medical possibilities) that may not even apply to your current complaints. Such information can create more anxiety, which you definitely do not need. In addition, when you self-diagnose as a patient, you decide on a medical diagnosis strictly based on your current or similar past symptoms, and you run the risk of arriving at the wrong diagnosis. You are also taking a chance of either underdiagnosing or over diagnosing your medical ailment. This is because similar symptoms may be evident in many different medical diagnosis, and without an actual clinician's assessment to further evaluate your symptoms and run appropriate tests, it is possible to miss other underlying medical problems that are initially not evident. The act of self-diagnosis can also be frowned upon by your clinician because it sometimes seems as though the patient who self-diagnoses undermines the role of the clinician. This perception does not promote the development of a productive clinician-patient relationship.

As listed in the do list, maintain a positive attitude with the clinic visit process. Endeavor to not display an inapproachable demeanor. It is much easier to smile at someone and get a smile in return than to maintain a frown on your face, which makes another person cautious in approaching you while he/she attempts to determine whether you are in a bad mood.

During the clinical consultation session, maintain your focus on the conversation regarding your clinical visit. Occasional social greetings to catch up with the clinician regarding your social and daily living routines since your previous visit is expected, but do not engage the clinician with nonclinical chitchat for extended periods of time. This creates unnecessary diversion and may distract the clinician from completely focusing on the clinical reason for your visit. Limit the use of electronic gadgets during clinical visit. Do not keep your head down, and don't check your electronic phones during clinical visits (especially while engaging in a clinical conversation with a clinician). It may be perceived as rude and dismissive by the clinician, and it does not promote a productive interaction.

Finally, don't be scared of the clinical visit experience. It is an empowering process designed to enable you to gain control of your health. A successful relationship with your clinician is a rewarding one that will help to keep you one step ahead of any impending disease. Over the years, I have found out that even when in doubt of a positive outcome with regard to the prognosis of a medical challenge, implementing these three important actions have tremendously helped me in coping with undesirable moments of life: "Laugh more than you cry, pray always, and remain optimistic." In addition to maintaining my regular visits with my clinicians and following the clinician's advice, I believe that these three principles contributed in helping me overcome my health challenges. They gave me the chance to return to my love of being an attentive clinician for my patients. As clinicians, we are instruments used by God to treat diseases, although God provides the ultimate healing of an individual. Whatever you are going through as a patient, it is vital that you never underestimate the power of prayers in your recovery process as you follow your clinician's recommendations. You will ultimately experience God's healing power.

Nonye Tochi Aghanya, MSc, RN, FNP-C

CHAPTER TWO
For Clinicians and Future Clinicians

Hello, clinicians. Who are you treating? The patient, or the disease? Or both?

I'm sure that many clinicians have heard these suggestions at some point: "Introduce yourself to a patient with a handshake, give a smile, maintain eye contact, and speak politely." As clinicians, we are under the impression that these are the vital requirements to achieve a productive consultation visit with a patient. Permit me to break that narrow-minded bubble! It is not entirely true. My past experiences interacting with patients for a thirty-year period have led me to realize that these positive attributes, although helpful, may not be all that are required of a clinician to achieve a productive consultation visit with every patient. It is vital that the clinician gain some awareness of the patient's personality traits and emotional status in order to more effectively relate with the patient.

To be noted is the importance of the clinician to examine her own values and attitudes prior to making patient contact each day. This brings to mind the popular sayings "I am not a morning person" and "I woke up on the wrong side of the bed." I have always believed that such statements are made on an attempt to excuse an individual's negative attitudes and behavior toward others. Clinicians, please know that in order to be effective in forming, developing, and maintaining relationships with your patients, you do not have the luxury to even think about such statements—or in worse cases, apply them in your daily practice—as a means to excuse an unreceptive mood on a difficult day with a patient.

However, I must note that it is unrealistic to expect every clinician to be in a pleasant or happy mood at all times. Let's face it: clinicians are still humans with real human emotions. (Although the clinician's ever- increasing daily workload can sometimes make one wonder whether there are some underlying supernatural powers that enable clinicians to achieve and maintain a decent amount of sanity with such hectic workloads!)

Clinicians, let me ask you this. When you first walk into a consultation room to meet with a new patient for the very first time, what do you typically think about? Naturally, most clinicians would think to themselves, "I hope the visit goes well with this patient." This is a normal human response because nobody wishes to leave a bad impression following a visit with another individual. Realistically, it doesn't always turn out that way. Although you try as hard as you can to leave a good impression, there would always be some patients who will not achieve a decent level of comfort in your presence to engage in an honest, productive conversation. This can become a deterrent to building a successful relationship.

Do you know that there is a strategic approach to experiencing a stress- free, successful, and productive consultation with each patient's visit that will ultimately result in trust improvement between clinicians and patients? The concept of clinician-patient communication has been discussed in various forums and remains a part of the curriculum in various health and medical educational institutions. However, the contents of this book will put a new spin on what you may already know about communicating with your patients. More often than not, effective communication between two individuals does not happen naturally at first. It must take a more conscious effort on the part of the clinician to be successfully achieved. It requires a skill that can be cultivated and improved when regularly applied over time by the clinician in several different scenarios. When the clinician invests time and effort to implement this approach, it becomes second nature and occurs more naturally and effortlessly, thus reducing the psychological stressors that are encountered with other methods for developing productive clinician-patient relationships. Several tips that are detailed in this book will help you, the clinician, develop the necessary skills that are needed to build and maintain a nurturing and rewarding relationship with your patients. Believe me, your patients will thank you.

Nonye Tochi Aghanya, MSc, RN, FNP-C

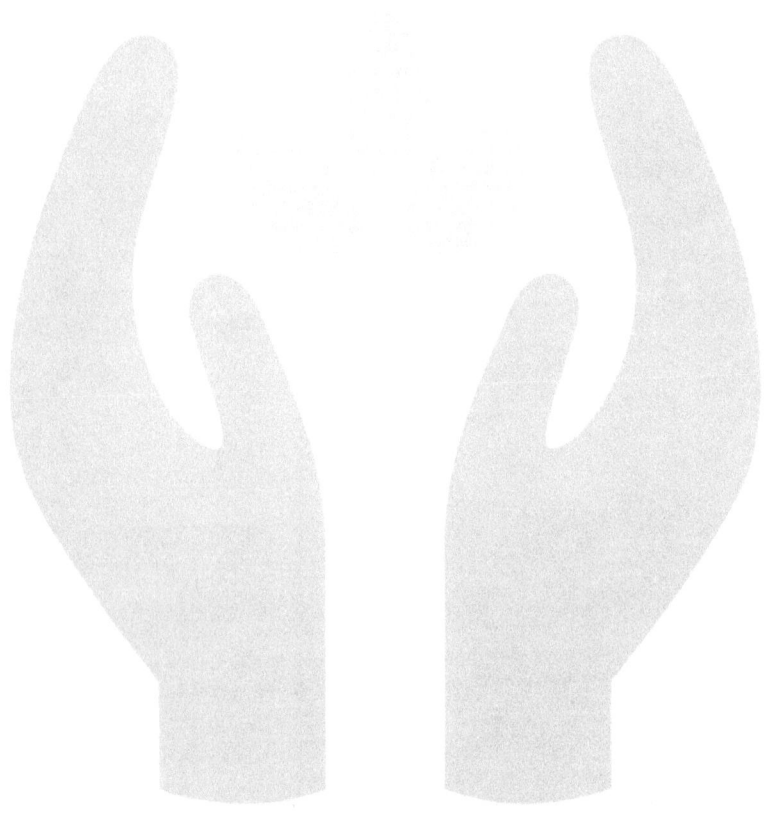

CHAPTER THREE
Talk to me, Doctor

It is no secret that all patients wish to be heard by their clinicians. But the question is "As a clinician, how do you know that a patient feels that he has heard and understood you following the consultation visit?"

A 2003 study report by T. Parkin and T. C. Skinner evaluated what patients remember after their visits with their health care providers. It examined whether patients and clinicians remembered what decisions were made following the consultation visits. They found out that in 50 percent of those clinic visits, there was substantial disagreement between patients' and clinicians' perceptions and recollections of the content of the consultation (Parkin and Skinner 2003).

It is important to note that the assessment reports of patient experiences are now being used to measure and report the quality of the clinician's care in all health care delivery settings such as hospitals, private medical practices, specialty care settings, home care, and retail care clinics. There are many diverse venues for patients to share their opinions, reviews, and online ratings. More than ever before, it seems as though the clinicians are under a microscope to meet the set standard of practice set by these governing bodies. The Hospital Consumer Assessment of Healthcare Providers and Systems (HCAHPS) survey is a standardized survey that allows for nationwide comparison of patient surveys. It is the standard by which hospitals, health systems, and individual hospitalists are judged.

The Center for Medicare and Medicaid Services (CMS) and the Agency for Health Research and Quality (AHRQ) developed and piloted a survey in 2002. They launched it in October 2006 and published the initial results in March 2008 on the Hospital Compare website. In this survey approach, there are several questions that capture the patient's general opinion regarding different aspects of the health care services. However, there are three questions that are more specific to clinician- patient interaction, and these focus on the quality of communication between the patient and the clinician. Let's take a look at these three questions and how they can be applicable to our own personal experiences with our patients. Although set in a hospital setting, it can be tailored and made applicable to other diverse specialties.

Question #1: During a hospital stay, how often did doctors treat you with courtesy and respect?

Question #2: During a hospital stay, how often did doctors listen carefully to you?

Question #3: During a hospital stay, how often did doctors explain things in a way you could understand?[1]

I can imagine that many of the patients who responded positively to these three questions are those who were completely their true selves while they were interacting with their doctors during their hospital stay. They felt that they were treated with respect, which helped them to become comfortable enough in the doctor's presence to voice their opinions. They believed their doctors listened to them. I've mentioned this earlier in the book, and it's worth repeating: the goal of every clinician should be to interact with patients when they are

---

[1] "Medicare Hospitals Compare Quality of Care," http://www.medicare.gov/hospitalscompare/About/Survey-Patients-experience.html. Accessed December 12, 2015.

their true selves. What exactly does it mean for someone to achieve a state of true self? This is accomplished when all barriers to communication (real and imagined) have been knocked down, and the patient's comfort level evolves to a point where the patient experiences less stress and anxiety, becomes less fearful, and has an honest state of mind while communicating with the clinician.

Over many years of interacting with patients, I have come to realize the two important factors that have helped my patients to quickly achieve a state of true self. First is a clinician's ability to feel empathy for the patient and demonstrate compassion. The next is a clinician's ability to communicate in a manner that assists the patient to become at ease in the clinician's presence. Several tips in developing these necessary skills are highlighted and discussed in detail in the subsequent chapters of this book. With repeated application of the required communication skills (both verbal and nonverbal), *all* clinicians possess the ability to assist their patients to become their true selves. The atmosphere of a consultation visit should be such that the patient is at an acceptable comfort level in order to absorb and retain the information discussed, such as current symptoms and differential diagnosis, applicable treatment options, the benefits of compliance, and the risks of noncompliance with treatment plans. When a patient has a pleasant experience at an initial visit with a clinician, the patient is more likely to be open, honest, and compliant with the clinician's recommendations during subsequent visits. This pattern is one that surely reduces the risk of medical malpractice and improves the clinician's job fulfillments.

In the new phase of health care management, which places much emphasis on clinical excellence, practice development, and clinician-patient survey reports, the utilization of electronic medical records for patients' consultations is more prevalent than ever before. As indicated earlier, the results of a recent survey that ranked the United States at number twenty-four is proof that with each passing year, more and more patients fail to make a genuine connection with their clinicians. Also, in such an emerging world where clinicians are required to adequately assess patients' histories, arrive at a diagnosis, and provide treatment in less time than previous years; it seems a more difficult task to rapidly establish a rapport with the patient while simultaneously accessing patient history and developing a treatment plan with patients. To be successful in building patient trust, the clinician must develop a unique approach to communicating with every patient. The clinician-patient relationship can be a simple or complex one depending on the clinician's approach to establishing an enduring relationship. It is unwise to assume that a productive clinician-patient relationship is achievable without much input from both parties. Just like every other relationship, there needs to be some effort made to develop and sustain the relationship so that it can be beneficial and fulfilling for both the clinician and the patient. Generally speaking, in order to ensure continued success, the clinician is expected to make more effort because the clinician is the authoritative figure who guides the flow of the consultation. Another error made by some clinicians is when they rely on patients to set the tone of a consultation visit and control the visit flow pattern.

However, many patients are expectantly looking to clinicians to set the tone of visits, and they are hopeful that it is a friendly and welcoming tone. Most patients will respond quickly and positively to a friendly tone from the clinician, and thus they would rather establish a rapport with the clinician than feel uncomfortable and fidget in the clinician's presence throughout the visit. Clinicians must take advantage of this common patient expectation and work with it in order to develop patient's trust. There is no disputing the fact that when people feel at ease, they retain more information disclosed to them.

Every individual has two types of memory: the cognitive and the emotional memory. Of these two types of memories, the emotional memory is more enduring. Maya Angelou characterized the distinction between these two types of memory when she eloquently and succinctly said, "I've learned that people will forget what you said, people will forget what you did, but people will never forget how you made them feel" (Sheppard 2015).

Cognitive Memory.
The prefrontal cortex plays an important role in cognitive control. Many previous studies have compared the functions of cognitive and emotional memory. These reports document the extensive research that have been conducted to examine cognitive control mechanisms for the selection and inhibition of responses, as well as selection of incoming sensory information. However, there is much less known about the selection of conceptual information or the selection of information in memory. From these reports, because emotional information receives priority in processing, there are many instances in which there is a need to exert control over the processing of (or the response to) such information. The concept of emotion regulation is considered critical to healthy emotional functioning and can be disrupted by a variety of different types of psychopathology. Lateral and medial prefrontal regions have been implicated in cognitive control relevant to emotions, such as suppressing the processing of emotional information or controlling emotional feelings. Cognitive control processes are the mechanisms through which humans use internal intentions to guide thought and behavior (Banich et al. 2009).

Emotional Memory.
Emotional experiences leave strong traces in the brain. Memories about emotional situations are stored in both the conscious and unconscious memory, which is part of the reason emotional memories are so enduring. Every new clinician should realize that patients often judge the quality of their medical care based on the emotion that they most experienced during their clinical interaction with the clinician. Many times, feelings of disconnect between clinicians and patients arise from the fact that clinicians live in their cognitive memories most of the time, whereas patients live in their emotional memories. There is nothing wrong with a clinician remaining objective and being cognitive with her approach to patient treatment; it is actually a critical skill that is necessary for efficient practice. Most clinicians are very conscious of this fact and

thus maintain a systematic discipline to keep personal feelings out of their minds during patient consultations. However, the downside is that some clinicians fall into a pattern of objectivity with all patient consultation sessions, without realizing that this creates a negative impact to the development of a productive relationship. It is important to note that a clinician must always maintain some level of emotional engagement with a patient in order for the consultation experience to be beneficial for both patient and clinician.

With my previous roles in various settings as a nurse's assistant, licensed practical nurse, registered nurse, and family nurse practitioner, I have come to realize that the process of establishing a meaningful relationship with a patient requires a delicate balancing act. My experiences in each role have prepared me to interact with patients in different scenarios with an exclusive approach that is applicable to that scenario, while considering the patient's traits and personalities. Patient personalities can alter the consultation environment in either a positive or a negative way. Regardless of a patient's personality (whether pleasant or unpleasant), the clinician should make every effort to apply the following four principles during each consultation session.

- First, acknowledge the patient's concern and seek out a point of agreement between you and the patient while establishing a tone for a respectful and successful conversation.
- Share some personal narrative (not too personal or intimate) about you as a clinician in order to make yourself relatable to the patient. This can help establish the patient's trust in your expertise, It may sometimes include a brief description of steps you've taken to build your knowledge base and expertise.
- Following your clinical assessment and medical decisions, briefly explain (without medical jargon) the scientific process behind your decision.
- Finally, offer advice to the patient based on that science.

Although all four principles steps will not be applicable to every patient consultation, many patients quickly become at ease in the clinician's presence, and patient trust in the clinician is improved when the clinician consistently applies most of these principles during consultations. Personally, I find that getting a good history from patients and then gently explaining physiological bodily activities resonates with patients, and they are more willing to accept their medical diagnosis, especially if the scientific evidence about their symptoms is presented in a way that they can understand and relate to. As a clinician, by taking the time to offer simple, clinical explanations to patients, you are validating the reality of the problem with them before proceeding with the subsequent steps of the clinical visit. Never underestimate the influence that your medical knowledge can have on your patients when disclosed in a relatable format. Always keep learning to stay up to date with evolving health practices and disease processes. *Never stop learning!*

Patient Adherence
Adherence to a healthy behavior pattern or lifestyle, as well as medication compliance, is difficult for most patients, especially for those who have cultivated poor behavioral habits over the years. Whether the clinician is addressing the patient's adherence to dietary patterns or keeping up with the patient regarding other habits that promote health, it is important for the clinician to understand that the process of trying to change patient behavior is a complex interplay between the patient, the clinician, and the health care system (Weber et al. 2015).

In reference to medication compliance, many years ago, it was easier for a clinician to observe that 65 percent of his patients on blood pressure medications were adherent to their regimen without the clinician having a clear understanding of the factors that contributed to such an observation. To get to the root of the issue of adherence, it is vital for clinicians to view patient adherence from the perspective of who initiated the behavior change or medical initiative, how well the patient executes the discussed regimen on a routine basis, and the patient's view on how a change in behavior or a new medication can affect her future plans. Unfortunately, many clinicians in previous years typically viewed adherence as strictly the patient's problem. Results of recent studies have proven that this is not the case. Patient behaviors are very much influenced by their perception of clinician input in their overall medical management plans.

An effective system of interaction typically involves numerous aspects of care. There should be scheduled follow-up phone calls from the clinician's offices, reminder brochures, periodic patient surveys, pleasant clinical practice environment, and more. These are only some of the many strategies that can positively influence patient behavior. No single strategy is likely to ensure a 100 percent patient adherence and behavior change but implementing one or more of these strategies will make a positive impact. Patients should be encouraged to ask questions about their diagnosis, the process of disease management, and medication importance, with emphasis placed on consequences and implications of nonadherence.

I know that at this point, many clinicians may be thinking, "But we do not have enough time to achieve this with each patient." I am in total agreement with that thought process! In recent times, it seems like with each subsequent year, clinicians are expected to do more in less time compared to previous years. This is why this book is a must-read for all clinicians, because the latter chapters contain details of several tips and guidelines that clinicians can apply in order to *improve the quality of time* spent with each patient while actually *reducing the quantity of time* spent during consultation visits. Various factors influence a patient's adherence, and a few of them involve the patient's emotional state of mind which may be evident in the patient's behavior pattern during consultation visits. It is vital for clinicians to pay close attention and ask questions regarding some of these factors: What are the underlying reasons for a patient's intentional lack of interest to implement medical plans? Is there a lack of social support and is the patient able to afford prescribed medications? What is the patient's anxiety level with regards to diagnosis and prognosis? Clinicians in various settings of practice can utilize a team approach system by including the nurse practitioners, office and medical assistants, dieticians, and social workers in the process of identifying and adequately addressing some of these factors, in order to improve patient adherence.

In developing information brochures for patients, the American Medical Association recommends that written health information should be targeted to a sixth-grade audience because nearly half of the US population is only marginally or functionally literate with an elementary or middle school reading level. This fact was noted in an online research report in the *American Journal of Surgery*. Per study findings, many patients leaving the hospitals do not understand follow-up care plans because the instructions are tailored to people with higher reading levels and more education (Choudhry et al. 2015). With knowledge of such information, clinicians can also conduct general surveys of their patients to ascertain average educational level and other interests that will assist in developing literature materials that are patient specific and easy to understand. Obtaining such knowledge gives the clinician more insight regarding the best approach to address the various factors that affect patient adherence.

Clinician-Patient Positioning
As a figure of authority, the clinician can unconsciously create an intimidating atmosphere when clinician-patient positioning is not considered an important factor. I am sure that all patients would prefer their clinicians speak to them rather than talk down at them. For the patient, the emotional recollection and the memory of the first consultation with a clinician is paramount in establishing trust. Clinicians should endeavor to maintain positions that patients would perceive as welcoming, nonthreatening, and not intimidating.

The aim is to establish horizontal eye contact between the clinician and the patient. In clinics where patient consultation is done with the patient sitting on the examination table, the clinician should stand by the examination table to maintain straight eye contact while communicating with the patient. If the clinician prefers to sit next to the examination table, a stool with a similar height as the exam table is the most appropriate option. Stools that are slightly lower in height than the exam table are also appropriate to use. If the patient is sitting down on a chair across from a clinician's desk, the clinician should sit on a chair of similar height. As much as possible, clinicians should avoid speaking to patients from a position that requires the patient's eye level to be significantly below that of the clinician's. Patients may perceive such a position as intimidating, with the assumption that the clinician is talking down at them rather than having a conversation with them. In the hospital setting, if the patient is lying down on the bed, the head of the bed should be slightly elevated during a visit with the clinician and the clinician should sit on a chair next to the bed.

When I was in the hospital recovering from my surgical procedure, I remember that my clinicians would sit by the edge of the bed while my head was elevated, and I always felt very appreciative that they didn't stand over my bed. When a clinician stands over a patient who is lying easily in bed, the towering figure of someone in an authoritative position can create feelings of anxiety, fear, and intimidation for a patient in such a dependent position. Although occasional clinician eye contact with the patient promotes acknowledgment, attentive listening is also very important. The clinician must not always maintain continuous eye contact with the patient at all times, in order to listen attentively. In some cultures, attentive listening and comprehension of the conversation content is better achieved when excessive eye contact is not maintained between both parties.

Clinicians should be aware of the factors that promote or hinder their individual listening skills. Observe the patient's body language. Most times, patients are reaching out for clinicians to make them feel at ease. Ask open-ended questions, and use teach-back methods with a shared decision-making process. Speak clearly and avoid excessive use of medical terminologies. Invite patient questioning and provide honest responses. Do not dismiss a patient's concerns. When you're not sure of a correct response, it's okay! Look it up in the literature, in the patient's presence. During my early years of practice as a clinician in pediatric and adult settings, I looked up information in my patient's presence and found that more patients appreciated clinicians that would make the effort to research and provide them with factual rather than made-up responses. Do not get into the habit of disclosing wrong information to patients in pretense. Medical knowledge is infinite. Never stop learning!

Use of Patient Information
To address patient confidentiality, two quotes from the American College of Physician Ethics manual sum it up well.

Confidentiality is a matter of respecting the privacy of patients, encouraging them to seek medical care and discuss their problems candidly, and prevent discrimination on the basis of their medical condition. The physician should not release a patient's personal medical information (often termed a privileged communication) without the patient's consent.

To uphold professionalism and protect patient privacy, clinicians should limit discussion of patient's and patient care issues to professional encounters. Discussion of patients by professional staff in public places, such as elevators, cafeterias violate confidentiality and is unethical. Outside of an educational setting, discussion of patients with or near persons who are not involved in the care of those patients impairs the public's trust and confidence in the medical profession. (Snyder 2012)

We can all agree that these two quotations seem to refer to protecting a patient's information in an era before the advanced digitalization of health care data. Thirty ago, when I started to interact with patients, there were none or very few social network sites. However, several literature and digital communication websites that provide clinicians with the option to post clinical opinions, seek comments, and share clinical views were in existence for many years before the Facebook and Twitter era. In recent years, with more advancements in the operation of networking sites and the increasing ease by which information can be transferred to large groups of individuals, some questions that must be addressed include "How much information is too much information to share?" and "Should patient consent be obtained prior to sharing clinical cases, even if the shared case studies do not reveal the patient's personal information?"

A study from a Medscape continuing medical education report brings this to light with a report about a resident who evaluated a patient that presented with a complaint of rashes. The patient's medical history showed her status was post breast augmentation. Her x-rays showed sarcoidosis, but her x-ray findings were partially obscured by the patient's breast implant. The consulting resident decided to post a picture that he took of the patient's rash on his Facebook page, and he also posted the patient's general history and test results. No personal information of the patient was disclosed in the Facebook post. The post received some comments about the breast implant, some of which were probably snickering remarks. The question of whether there is a breach of ethics and professionalism comes to mind in this scenario. This can be debated on so many different levels, based on each debater's perspective of right and wrong conduct (Snyder and Tilburt 2016).

It is noteworthy to remember that in this digitalized age, all clinicians must display professional judgment with reference to the transfer of patient's medical reports. Although the resident in the above case report did not disclose the patient's personal information, clinicians should always keep in mind that public perception of the clinician's conduct is vital to the development of patient's trust in the health care system. Clinicians should note that they are bound to a higher behavior standard than the general public because such a standard contributes to fostering a long-term, productive clinician-patient relationship. Facebook is a public social network space visible to an unlimited number of individuals. By posting such a report on Facebook, this resident had a well-intended purpose of sharing medical knowledge with fellow colleagues while gathering differential diagnoses and comments. But he lacked the judgment of not using a more restricted medical online site to submit his clinical set and seek opinions. Various online sites designed with the intention of promoting the sharing of clinical knowledge among clinicians have emerged in recent years, some with state identification requirements and security restrictions that encourage patient consent. Through these sites, clinicians can safely review submitted cases, and they can also submit clinical cases for review while minimizing the risk of public input and perceptions. An example of such service is Figure 1 Inc., with a website and a free downloadable application that clinicians and other individuals can access in order to share various medical contents and picture images for teaching and learning purposes. As of August 2016, Figure 1 Inc. listed on its website that this service is available in over one hundred countries.

Nonye Tochi Aghanya, MSc, RN, FNP-C

CHAPTER FOUR

Hello, Patient ... but Who Are You?

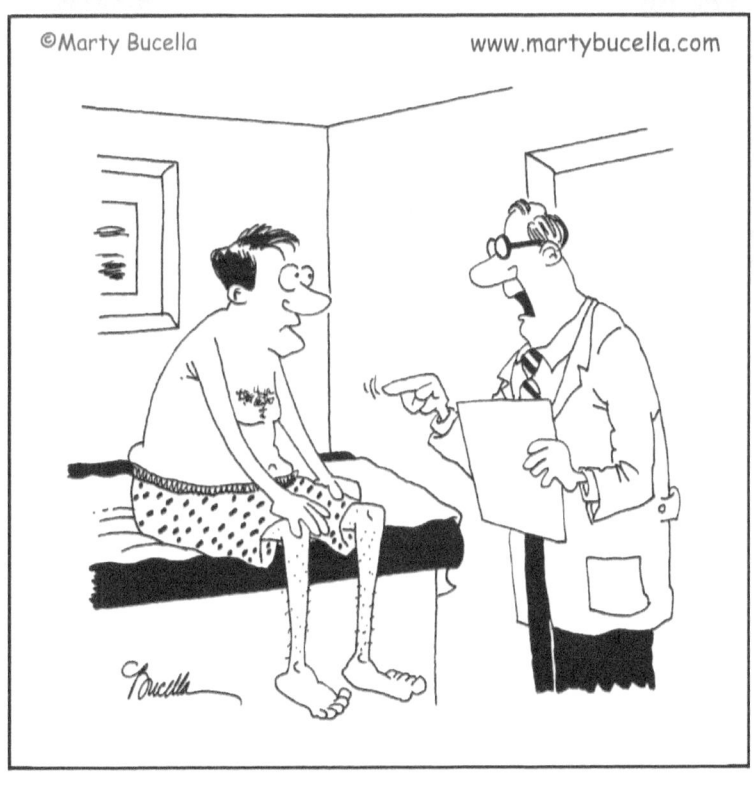

Nonye Tochi Aghanya, MSc, RN, FNP-C

The general consensus is that how we clinicians relate to patients is based on the knowledge we have about the patient, or who we perceive the patient to be. This information (real or perceived) enables us, as clinicians, to come up with targeted conversational topics that will help the consultation unfold successfully. Realistically, as much as we hate to admit it, we develop our perceptions of other groups of individuals based on what we have heard about those groups, based on what we've read or the media's portrayal of other groups. It is unproductive and unfair to relate to other groups of individuals solely based on our perceptions of them. More often than not, these are inaccurate and narrow perceptions. How you relate to a person is based on what you know or think you know about the person. In order to be an effective clinician, you must take the time to know your patients. It is a necessity.

In Dr. H. Gilbert Welch's book *Less Medicine, More Health*, he narrated a very interesting story of a new patient that he treated for elevated blood sugar, which was discovered during the patient's routine physical examination and blood test review. He mentioned that the blood sugar medication (oral hypoglycemic agent, or OHA) that he initiated on this patient may have "worked too well" in lowering the patient's blood sugar because this ultimately contributed to a hypoglycemic episode with devastating effects. In this very well-written book, Dr. Welch fast- forwarded to fifteen years of having open communication and more in- depth interactions with this patient (by taking time to really know the patient). Later on, he realized that the patient did not even need the OHA in the first place. He also noted that in all the subsequent years after he discontinued the oral medication for blood sugar control, the patient did not develop any symptoms or complications from the disease. This is because, as he stated in his book, he "got to know the patient well." He took the time to interact and develop a productive clinician-patient relationship. He discussed the patient's family, sports, and interests with him. In his book, Dr. Gilbert Welch wittingly summarizes that the focus for best health practice and medical management should be on learning about the patient and promoting patient health in ways that fit the patient's approach to life (Welch 2015, 108–111).

With the average clinician's workload comprising of an approximately twenty-five patients or more per day, it may seem like an uphill battle to achieve this. It is also an intricate task, given the various patient personalities that the clinician encounters daily. As a clinician, you may be asking yourself, "How can I get to know the true patient?" First and foremost, examine your own traits. Undergoing a process of introspection will help you as a clinician to know who you are, what your beliefs are, what your expectations of a patient are, what easily agitates or irritates you, and what level of patience you can exercise when confronted with an annoying behavior. It helps you determine what characteristics and values you admire most in other individuals (kindness, boldness, tenacity, shyness, timidity, nonchalance, fearlessness, compassion, etc.). This introspective process will also help you determine whether you are a compassionate person, or whether you get easily irritated when things are not going as you planned. Most importantly, it will help you examine how you respond to different individuals with diverse traits and personalities that are different from yours. I am not a psychiatrist but following my interactions with so many patients over the years, I believe that we all have various levels of social and moral values that are inherent in all of us. With time, our interactions with others may influence our judgment and behaviors.

In addition, based on environmental and social impacts that we are exposed to, as well as our individual life experiences, we consciously or unconsciously gravitate toward those values and characteristic that will eventually become more dominant in our lives. While I researched materials for this book, I also did a self-reflection of my own values and tried to identify the extent that my values influence the interactions I have with patients. The result of careful reflection revealed a common trait I possess that has enabled me to successfully develop an honest, productive relationship with each of my patients regardless of a patient's diverse values and characteristics. I believe I inherited compassion from my mother.

Thanks, Mom! The ability for a clinician to genuinely demonstrate compassion is 50 percent of the battle won.

What is compassion? According to *Merriam-Webster's Dictionary*, "Compassion is a feeling of wanting to help someone who is sick, hungry, in trouble, etc. It is a sympathetic consciousness of others' distress together with a desire to alleviate it" (*Merriam-Webster's* 2003). The key word is *feeling*. To be a proficient clinician, you must embark on developing a compassionate approach to health care management. This book is a guide for obtaining simple tips to assist the clinician identify, understand, and effectively relate to diverse patient traits and personalities in various health care settings. With illustrations and sample clinician-patient dialogues, several tips to developing the skills needed for effective communication are disclosed in each chapter. These skills are easy to acquire with appropriate effort. Take, for instance, the nurse-patient relationship. Nurses have a reputation for being angels of mercy. This is because nurses do the simple, empathetic gestures that let patients know they are being cared for. These feelings endure in the patients' memories long after treatment is over.

Clinicians should recognize that even though patients sometimes make attempts to hide their feelings, many patients experience anxiety and are usually more reserved during the initial consultation visits. Unfortunately, on some occasions, clinicians do not recognize these feelings of anxiety and are so focused on the cognitive memory that they neglect to address the patient's fear lurking under the surface. When a clinician takes a few minutes to acknowledge a patient's emotions and reassures the patient that the clinician is compassionate toward the patient's current predicament, it creates a lasting impact on the patient and goes a long way toward improving clinician-patient relationships. This simple demonstration of compassion by the clinician makes the patient recognize that in addition to making the effort to address the patient's symptoms, the clinician also cares for the patient's feelings. This is a crucial step to initiating an honest communication pattern and building a productive relationship with the patient. Remember the concept of *true self*? This is also a necessary step toward assisting a patient become his or her true self.

As stated earlier, if this process of displaying genuine compassion is implemented successfully, half the battle of achieving a productive clinician-patient relationship is won. The other 50 percent of the battle is all about the clinician's ability to identify a patient's personality and must respond appropriately in a manner that assists the patient to feel at ease in the clinician's presence. Patients who feel at ease during their consultation with a clinician are more compliant with recommended treatment plans as they begin to cultivate a sense of not wanting to let the clinician down with each subsequent visit. The clinician's ability to accurately interpret and appropriately respond to diverse patient personalities is developed over time. With repeated application of the guidelines and tips in this book that help to reduce patient anxiety, this ability becomes perfected until it feels like second nature. As time progresses, it becomes easier for the clinician to apply the appropriate verbal and nonverbal communication skills to specific patient scenarios with successful results.

In all my years of interacting with patients of diverse personalities (and heaven knows there are plenty of patient personalities in existence!), I've realized that in order to achieve a productive result with patient interaction, each patient's personality demands a specific clinical style of approach that is effectively applicable to that personality. To determine the appropriate style of interaction, the clinician must first determine what the patient's personality is. Thus, I have narrated in this book sixteen styles of interaction based on a clinical scenario and the patient's personality type. There could be more types of personalities out there in the world, but these are the ones that I've most often come across with in my years of interacting with patients. The following chapters of this book explore each patient personality, identify common traits of patients with such personalities (their common fears, communication weaknesses, and strengths), and disclose how the clinician can apply the necessary communication skills (verbal and nonverbal) to address communication obstacles and ultimately break communication barriers in order to establish a successful clinician-patient relationship. Only when this is achieved can a clinician unequivocally admit that the clinician has treated both the patient and the presenting disease.

CHAPTER FIVE

The Angry Patient

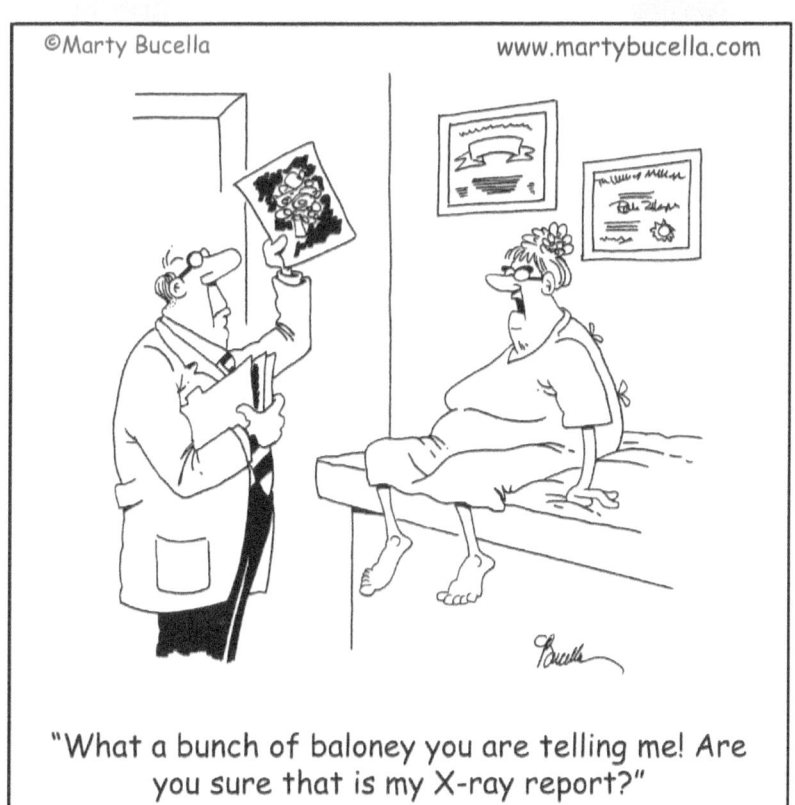

"What a bunch of baloney you are telling me! Are you sure that is my X-ray report?"

As a clinician, you will occasionally encounter an angry patient in your practice. There are various reasons (real and imagined) why patients become angry and deem it justifiable to display anger towards a clinician. Regardless of a patient's perceived reasons for being angry, the clinician usually does not have any control over a patient's choice to display behaviors that reveal underlying anger. However, as a clinician, you do have some control over your own actions to defuse a patient's emotions of anger and minimize the chances of escalating a confrontation. It is also important to note that clinicians have the necessary communication skills (verbal and nonverbal) to effectively interact with the angry patient while making it a positive learning experience for both the clinician and the patient.

In the practice of medicine, one interesting thing that I've observed over the years is that anger is not always a negative emotion. At least, that's the perspective I've consciously decided to take as I approach and interact with an angry patient. Although it's easily viewed by many as a negative emotion, my observation is that anger is actually the emotion that affords patients the ability to readily tap into their most vulnerable state and thus disclose their most truthful thoughts and feelings without much reservation. Patients may have a perspective of a situation that is different from the clinician's, and this could either be positive or negative, real or imagined. When patients are angry, they tend to easily disclose what's on their minds without regard to their perspective of the situation. I've realized that when patients display emotions of anger during consultation visits, it is not uncommon for clinicians to avoid having detailed conversations with the patient, or they get offended and sometimes become confrontational as the clinician attempts to divert from exploring the origin of such anger. However, if harnessed properly, this raw emotion of anger that affords the angry patient the ease to speak freely is very vital in developing an honest, productive relationship between the clinician and the patient.

Many years ago, prior to my realization of the effective strategy for communicating with an angry patient, I struggled to find the best approach to communicate with such a patient while maintaining my professionalism and limiting the chances of being provoked. I realized many years later in clinical practice that as a new clinician, I probably needed to experience those encounters with an angry patient because such encounters afforded me the opportunity to improve my ability to listen, maintain composure, and exercise patience with a patient who was upset and not seemingly nice to me. It also enabled me to observe patients in their vulnerable states (the closest state to a true self). The interesting thing is that many patients who interact with clinicians while angry may not realize that they are close to displaying their true selves. This is because an angry patient does not have any reservations about speaking his or her mind, and clinicians can benefit from getting the most truthful responses to the questions posed to such a patient. I have found that my consultations with the angry patient have helped me implement accurate medical plans and productive measures for the patient's benefit.

Many patients who are angry may not initially engage the clinician in a dialogue. They may tend to initially internalize their emotions and may only provide yes or no responses to the clinician's questions. When such anger further erupts into a raw emotion, patients tend to make more verbal responses with an unfriendly attitude as they open up and provide more information. It is important for the clinician to ignore the anger and apply appropriate communication skills in order to develop a productive clinician-patient dialogue.

As a clinician, how do you know that you are dealing with an angry patient? The first indication that you may have an angry patient on your hand is the patient's blatant resistance and disregard of your clinical suggestions. Typically, such patients have no qualms verbalizing that resistance to you. An angry patient may be very rude and confrontational. Some patients are downright oppositional and may even make inappropriate and unprofessional statements. Many years ago, I once had a patient angrily say to me, "If you don't know what you are doing, maybe you should just step down and let someone who knows the job take over." This statement was made following the administration of a flu vaccination after which the patient experienced a very sore spot at the site of injection. Of course, this patient probably did not know that there is an up to 64 percent chance of experiencing soreness at an injection site for adults and children following the intramuscular administration of a flu vaccine. In addition, the patient may not have known that there are measures that can be implemented to reduce these chances (Brown 2016).

When a patient angrily utters such a statement to a clinician (especially one who has just provided medical care to the patient), it is a natural human response for the clinician to feel insulted, unappreciated, or even angry. However, harboring such feelings will only encourage the clinician to put up a defensive wall, which can further deter effective communication between the clinician and the patient as the visit progresses. When I encountered such a scenario, I immediately took a different approach and reflected on the fact that the patient was not aware of the statistics regarding flu vaccination and injection sites. Rather than feel insulted or upset, I felt an obligation to inform this patient that it was not uncommon to experience soreness at injection sites. I also disclosed the different measures that could be taken to reduce the chances of such occurrence in the future. I informed the patient of measures such as "avoiding making tight muscles or fists during the injection; resting the arm and avoiding exercises that isolates the biceps, triceps, and deltoid muscles for at least twenty-four hours post-vaccination and taking Tylenol or Advil as needed after the vaccination."

This patient was very appreciative of the information I offered and seemed surprised that I was not offended! For the rest of the consultation, I noticed that the patient made an effort to be courteous and kind while communicating with me. By consciously making sure that the patient did not perceive me as becoming upset or defensive in response to a statement made in anger (instead viewing me as a source of information), I reduced my chances of experiencing feelings of humiliation, anger, embarrassment, or hurt. I reversed the intent of the patient's angry emotion and maintained the authority as the clinician by being the educator, and I provided the patient with information to alleviate future occurrences.

This approach, which I've implemented for the past thirty years, has always been effective in my encounters with the angry patient. It is the principle approach to effective communication with such a patient. Although the above example is a simple one regarding vaccination and adverse events, this approach is also effective in all scenarios that involve patients who are disrespectful or condescending, and who display emotions of anger toward the clinician. The clinician should feel empowered with the fact that clinical knowledge has the propensity to turn a negative into a positive and can diffuse a confrontational situation when this knowledge is gently presented in a simple and targeted format.

When confronted by an angry patient, it is important for the clinician to maintain focus on the communication approach, and to refrain from interrupting while the patient is speaking. The clinician should pay close attention to determine the accuracy of the patient's statements. Sometimes, the patient's clinical assumptions may be reliable medical facts, but in many cases, the assumptions are only partially correct because patients tend to obtain medical information from less reliable sources such as websites, social networks, and friends and families. As a new clinician, don't be alarmed if you encounter patients who would pull out their iPhones in the midst of a clinical conversation and search various sites to verify information you've provided to them during the consultation. Given your knowledge base and clinical skills, it becomes your responsibility as the patient's clinician to offer more evidence-based medical information while correcting any wrong assumptions that the patient may have.

From my past experiences, this technique is a proven recipe for success in reducing patient anxiety and anger, and in ultimately defusing a potentially confrontational scenario. I have learned not to implement the following techniques, which deter effective communication: becoming angry, confrontational, or condescending when responding to the angry patient; pretending that I did not hear the patient's statement; and completely ignoring the patient. These used to be my approaches as a new clinician until I realized that they were counterproductive in building an honest clinician-patient relationship. Patients may interpret a clinician's confrontational response or total lack of response as uncaring behavior, and that can only escalate the patient's anger, ultimately resulting in total communication breakdown.

CHAPTER SIX

The Opinionated (Overly Confident) Patient

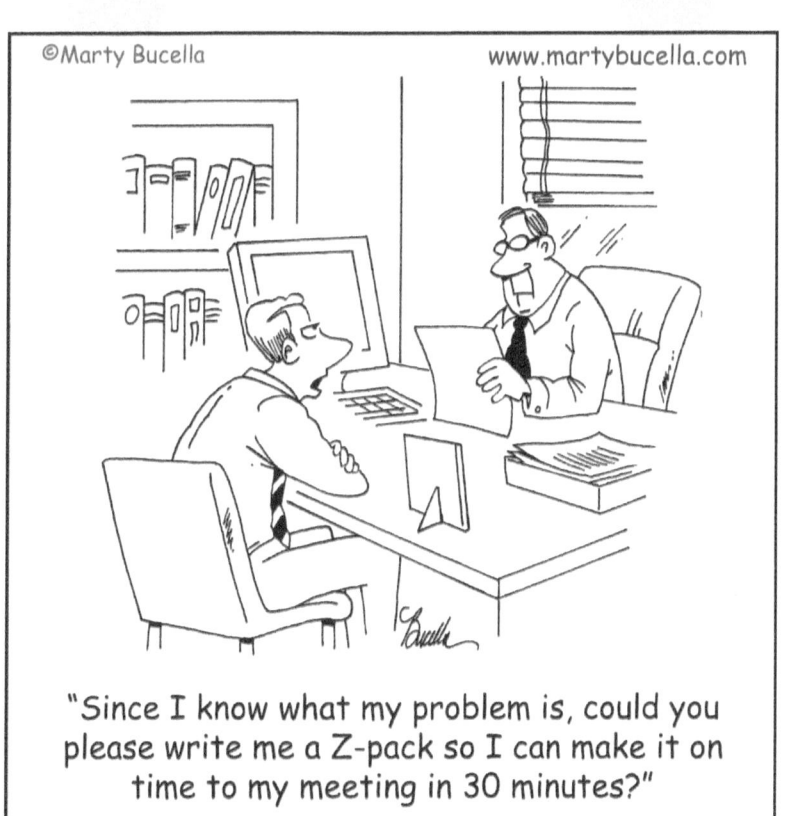

"Since I know what my problem is, could you please write me a Z-pack so I can make it on time to my meeting in 30 minutes?"

Many clinicians may not readily admit this, but ask yourself a question: Have you ever come across a patient whose mannerisms made you feel rushed or uncomfortable? I have experienced such feelings in my years of clinical practice. As clinicians, we encourage patients to embark on lifestyle changes and participate in activities that would improve health, build confidence, and improve social and communication skills. We all know that these are qualities that reduce an individual's chances of becoming a victim of life's circumstances, and all clinicians would prefer that their patients have a good sense of healthy confidence. Confidence is knowing what you're good at, understanding the value you provide, and acting in a way that conveys it to others. This is different from arrogance (which I also equate to being overly confident), which involves erroneously believing that you are better in a particular area than you actually are. But when does confidence become too much confidence? Unfortunately, one can display a false sense of high confidence that gradually progresses to arrogance. This is a characteristic that is often displayed by the opinionated patient.

At some point in your clinical practice, you will come across the opinionated patient. This is the patient who displays an unhealthy level of confidence in his or her medical knowledge and the ability to interpret signs and symptoms of diseases that may impact compliance with appropriate treatment plans. It is not uncommon for opinionated patients to verbalize to the clinician that they know the most appropriate medical course of action to implement for their health management. Another identifier (although it's not always specific) could be a patient who prefers to stand during a consultation and look down at a sitting clinician, rather than sit in the empty seat by the clinician. Such a patient may also prefer to be examined in a standing position rather than on the examination table. The clinician should not encourage such behavior by examining the patient while the patient is in a standing position, especially if there exists a high risk of patient falls (e.g., while administering vaccinations or performing certain neurological exams). It is important for the clinician to gently ask the patient to sit down. The general positioning guidelines detailed in chapter 3 should be implemented to assist the patient to feel more at ease in the clinician's presence.

The opinionated patient is typically well-versed with easy access to medical literature and materials. He or she stays up-to-date with the evolving health care system. With time, however, this amassed body of health knowledge creates a high level of confidence, which the patient erroneously interprets as a license to dictate and direct the clinician regarding treatment plans. Quite frankly, of all the patient categories that are highlighted in this book, the opinionated patient may be the most difficult with whom to easily cultivate an honest, trusting relationship. This is because such a patient strongly believes in the saying "I know my body, so I know what I need." Effective communication with such a patient is achievable with the application of specific communication (verbal and nonverbal) guidelines.

The main goal of a clinician is to gently but firmly persuade acceptance of a medical plan by exploring various treatment options with every patient. Do not totally dismiss the patient's views. There is no one way to do this because it can be achieved in various ways. Over the years, I've realized that it is more easily achievable when a clinician has a strong clinical knowledge base and implements a decisive mannerism in the communication technique. What do I mean by such a statement? In this chapter, I will give some instances of my encounters with opinionated patients and the communication patterns that have enabled me to better communicate and develop a trusting relationship.

It is not very difficult to identify the opinionated patient. This patient usually researches and obtains medical knowledge from reliable (or sometimes unreliable) sources, citing such references while questioning the clinician's decisions during consultations. There are also patients who may have chronic medical conditions for which they've had repeated visits to several specialty doctors. These patients are typically fully aware of their previous treatment plans from these various specialists and they sometimes emphatically emphasize to the clinician that such plans must be implemented during consultation.

A Case of Lupus Flare-Up?

Many years ago, I had a fifty-year-old patient, whom I'll refer to as "Mrs.
M." She had a past medical history of lupus since she was twenty years of age. She presented with complaints of an upper respiratory infection and cold symptoms. Early in the consultation, she sat upright in her chair, and with a straight back and a very steady eye contact with me, she remarked sharply, "I know that this is not my lupus acting up, because with that, I always get a fever and a rash. I just have a cold and I need antibiotics." If you are a new clinician, a patient's seemingly confident posture, coupled with the fact that she's had lupus for many years and knows her body well, this may make you lean more toward considering her suggestions, and it may incite self-doubt in your own clinical judgment. But don't forget that as a clinician, even if it initially appears that a patient is very knowledgeable about her chronic disease, she may sometimes be misinformed with regards to an acute illness presentation.

As the clinician, you possess the skills to communicate effectively with the patient and persuade the acceptance of your plan of care based on your current assessment and findings. Listen to the patient's statements. Acknowledge the correct aspects of the patient's statement, but emphasize to the patient in a calm, authoritative, and non-confrontational tone that there are other aspects of the disease process (which the patient may not be familiar with) that could be overlooked when disease management is solely based on the patient's perspectives. Good communication skills can effectively persuade acceptance. In the above scenario with Mrs. M, I said, "You are correct about fever and rash as signs of lupus flare-up, but there are also other subtle signs that may not be as evident. This is why I prefer we run some blood tests to ensure that we look at the whole clinical picture and do not miss anything."

Notice that I use the word we while suggesting my clinical recommendations. I have found the use of such statements very effective in relaying to the opinionated patient that as the clinician, you are making a medical decision based on several factors that include the patient's reported history and your medical expertise. Clinical management is a joint venture between you and the patient, and all patients (especially the opinionated patients) appreciate that their perspective is included in the medical decision-making process. Although you do not wish to discredit any information provided by the patient regardless of the manner of presentation, you should always aim to direct the flow of the clinical visit and maintain control of the suggested and initiated treatment plans.

A Case of Leg Pains?

Another scenario was a clinical visit I had with a sixty-year-old man, whom I'll refer to as "Mr. X." He came to the clinic with complaints of right ankle pain. During the history exam, "Mr. X" narrated that he experienced some leg pains following a game of golf two days prior to his visit. He wasn't sure if he'd sustained any injury while playing golf but said he firmly believed he'd sprained his ankle as he bent down to strike the golf ball. Mr. X seemed very irritable and was not focused or easily forthcoming with responses to the questions I asked during the history-taking process. Rather, he continued to state that he believed this was simply an ankle sprain. He kept glancing at his watch as though he wanted to rush the visit along.

At this point, I momentarily stopped asking him questions. Rather, I listened as he spoke for a while, giving several other reasons why he believed this was an ankle sprain. Many clinicians will agree that such a scenario can be very distracting (and sometimes annoying) when a patient becomes fixated on a self-diagnosis and refuses to provide more history that can assist in exploring other differential diagnosis. However, there are simple guidelines to establishing an effective communication with the opinionated patient who presents in this manner. First, the clinician should not engage in an adversary debate with the patient, especially in the initial minutes of the conversation even if the clinician is not in agreement with the patient's opinion.

In the scenario with Mr. X, I deliberately did not maintain steady eye contact with him, but intermittently glanced at him as he spoke while I wrote down notes. I occasionally nodded my head to establish the fact that I was listening to his points. After a few minutes, I noticed Mr. X's demeanor gradually change from an irritable to calm demeanor as he continued speaking. He glanced at his watch less frequently, and his tone of voice was less demanding. Please note that this non-confrontational approach of providing assurance to the patient that the clinician is listening while giving the patient some time to verbalize his opinions creates an atmosphere of tranquility that helps diminish the patient's anxiety and contributes to establishing a trend of behavior changes. With this approach, I have found that such a patient exhibits reduced irritability as the patient becomes less fixated on a pattern of self-diagnosis and gradually begins to explore other contributory factors.

Also in this scenario with Mr. X; as I listened and took notes, he proceeded to tell me that his right leg and calf had been slightly swollen two weeks prior to his visit. But he didn't think that it was a big deal because he did not experience pain until two days ago following his golf game. This prompted me to do a Doppler study in addition to an x-ray of the right leg and ankle. The result showed that Mr. X did not have a fracture or a sprain, but a deep vein thrombosis. He was quite grateful for my patience and thanked me immensely. He made sure he followed up with me periodically as we explored (with the hematology specialist) the etiology and other possible contributory factors to the development of his thrombus.

Each time I reflect back on that scenario, I remember exactly what helped me to initiate the most appropriate treatment plan for his complaint. Despite the initial communication difficulties with Mr. X, the key to finally establishing a trusting relationship was to avoid being confrontational or creating an atmosphere of intimidation with the use of medical jargon. This is counterproductive because it can elicit defensive characteristics in the patient, which in turn become a deterrent for the clinician in getting to know the patient's true feelings and concerns. I did not appear timid or overstate safety to Mr. X. I used simple, factual medical descriptions while communicating with him. It is important for the clinician to appear confident, calm, and in control of the visit when communicating with the overly confident patient.

A Case of the Flu?

During the month of July, a nine-year-old boy visited the clinic with his mother. He had symptoms of rhinitis and cough for about one week. I will refer to the mother as "Mrs. Y." While I sat at my desk, Mrs. Y came into the clinic and stood over me while the nine-year-old patient sat on the examination table. Take note that rather than sit in the empty chair across the desk from me, Mrs. Y preferred to stand as she narrated her son's medical history. She stated that her son had the flu about two years ago, and his current symptoms were similar to the symptoms he had two years ago. She asked that I prescribe some Tamiflu for her son so that she could leave on time in order to make it to her next engagement. As she stood over me and spoke, I could sense her rising anxiety, and there was increasing tension in the environment. After I completed taking history notes, I stood up and gently walked over to her son on the exam table.

While examining the patient, Mrs. Y casually mentioned that she was concerned that she may have contracted the flu from her son because she'd developed a cough about four days ago. She further said she had just concluded a board meeting earlier that day. When I heard this, I saw that this was a perfect opportunity to establish better communication and reduce parent anxiety. I said, "Wow, how was the meeting? I hope you didn't cough a lot. Talking typically induces coughing spells for most people." She smiled and said she had the cough under control because she intermittently sipped water from a bottle she had during the meeting. "Okay," I said to her, "but don't forget that you can come back to the clinic to be examined for that cough if it gets any worse." Following that very minor conversation, she seemed a bit more relaxed, walked over to the empty chair and sat down as I proceeded to complete her son's physical examination.

Following my assessment, I informed her that the findings did not suggest her son had the flu, but rather an upper respiratory viral infection. I informed her of the reasons I didn't believe her son had the flu: July was not flu season, her son's symptoms had lingered for about seven days, and it was not of a sudden onset in nature. She listened attentively without opposition, and I had an engaging conversation with her about the differences between influenza viral symptoms and other viral presentations. I truly believe I was able to accomplish this because I took the time to have a very brief conversation regarding her statement about her own minor cough symptoms. She felt that I cared enough to inquire about the impact her cough had earlier in the day during her meeting. Sometimes, all a clinician needs to do is simply verbalize one or two appropriate statements that show concern in order to reduce a parent's anxiety and make a connection. Considering the benefits of such action, that is not a difficult task at all to initiate. Mrs. Y's son was prescribed a cough expectorant, some analgesics, and a nasal wash. He recovered completely within a few days.

Sometimes, the clinician needs to find a point of interest for a brief conversation with the anxious patient or the parent of a minor in order to break the ice. To achieve the most effective consultation, this is usually an important step to implement before the clinician proceeds to explain the medical findings, possible disease etiology, and clinical suggestions. When this is not accomplished, many patients, in their state of discomfort or anxiety may become overly analytical of the clinician's suggestions or may pay little or no attention to the clinician's suggestions. It is the clinician's responsibility to assist the patient in feeling at ease with the consultation visit.

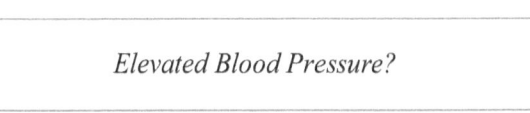

Elevated Blood Pressure?

Many years ago, while I worked in my private clinic where I monitored patients who were on blood thinners, I had a fifty-year-old patient whom I will refer to as "Mr. Z." The patient was taking a blood thinner, *Coumadin*, and arrived to check the level of his international normalized ratio (INR). The visit proceeded smoothly until I checked his blood pressure and noticed that it was elevated, at 150/94. I informed Mr. Z that I needed to monitor his blood pressure closely, or he should see his primary care doctor or cardiologist within one week for reassessment. He immediately became upset and told me that he did not have high blood pressure. He seemed more irritated as I further attempted to explain the consequences of being on blood thinners with high blood pressure (risks of hemorrhagic stroke, bleeding aneurysms, etc.). I also attempted to discuss some dietary changes that he needed to make that would help lower his blood pressure. At this point, Mr. Z appeared more agitated as he sharply remarked,

"I don't know why you are pushing this issue. I told you that I do not have high blood pressure. I always get my yearly physicals at my doctor's and have never been told that I have high blood pressure."

When I realized that my current approach to establishing a productive communication with him was not effective, I decided to switch my approach. I calmly asked, "So what do you do for a living?" He said that he was a middle school coach and had just completed coaching a game within the past twenty-four hours. "Oh, that explains it, then!" I remarked with an amused expression on my face. "I can only imagine the effort required of you to remain pleasant with the parents who probably think that their kids are the best players on the team. I'm sure it's not uncommon for parents to argue with you and with one another. That's enough stress to elevate anyone's blood pressure, including mine!" Mr. Z laughed out loud and said that I was correct. Once I observed that I had assisted him to feel more at ease, I then repeated my earlier recommendations for closer blood pressure monitoring because of his regular involvement in such a highly competitive, charged atmosphere. I asked him to keep a weekly self- monitoring log of his blood pressure levels and return to me or follow up with his primary care doctor in one week. At this suggestion, Mr. Z smiled broadly, thanked me, and said that he would definitely do so.

This scenario drives home the point that the clinician should refrain from becoming upset with a patient who initially disagrees with the clinician's observations and suggestions. An alternate approach is to find a means (in the case with Mr. Z, humor) to lower the patient's defenses and improve patient reception. Once achieved, the clinician should again present the clinical recommendations.

CHAPTER SEVEN
The Dependent Patient

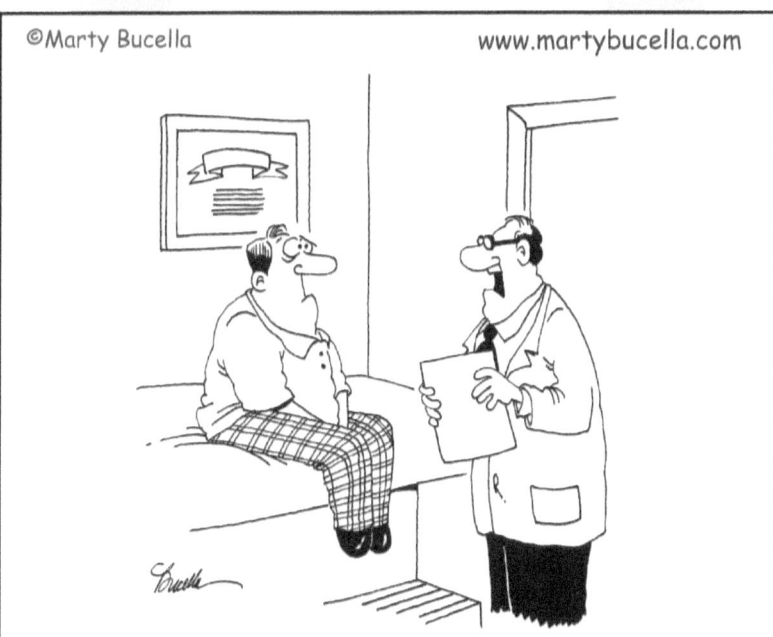

"Your heart, blood pressure and cholesterol are fine, but I'm concerned with the way you stare without saying much. Do you have any questions?"

The dependent patient typically relies completely on the clinician's judgment and suggestions while making little or no effort to contribute to the dialogue. I have noticed that a patient may not present as a dependent patient on initial consultation visits, but sometimes with subsequent visits, the patient's perceptions of the clinician's general response, attitude, and behavior may contribute to a patient's gradual transition into dependence. A really bad scenario is when a clinician's actions or inactions contribute to transforming an angry or opinionated patient into a dependent patient. A sure enough way to make that happen is when clinicians ignore a patient's concerns and suggestions during consultations. When a patient's concern is ignored, the patient may begin to view the interaction as a one-sided dialogue, and if the patient experiences the same communication pattern with subsequent visits, he or she may develop a reservation and timidity about voicing opinions during future visits. At some point, the patient may even deem it as being rude for him or her to voice opinions to the clinician about treatment plans and other concerns. Such assumptions may turn a patient into one who then totally depends on the clinician's judgment and suggestions.

The difference between the dependent patient and the opinionated patient is that this patient is usually not critical of the clinician's clinical suggestions. Another factor that may contribute to patient dependency is the patient's underlying traits and personality. In such cases, this nature of patient dependency is not necessarily a result of the clinician's impact on the patient. The innate personality may be of a cultural or psychological basis. An underlying concern that many dependent patients have is an unsubstantiated fear of upsetting the clinician by asking questions. Regardless of how friendly, nice, and welcoming a clinician may appear, the dependent patient will always find a reason to put up a wall because of fear of upsetting the doctor by asking too many questions. This patient has a tendency to nod affirmatively in response to all the clinician's questions and rarely gives information or asks questions when prompted. Even when the patient's lifestyle will not accommodate a clinical plan initiated by the clinician, the dependent patient will not inform the clinician but would rather leave a consultation with the knowledge that such clinical plans will not be implemented. Instead of verbalizing reservations or restrictions to implementing a clinical plan so that alternate measures can be discussed, the patient would rather feel more comfortable by remaining quiet or responding to all questions with simple yes or no responses. The clinician then wrongly assumes that an appropriate medical plan has been initiated—and becomes surprised when the patient does not effectively respond to the plan.

During an encounter with the dependent patient, the goal is for the patient to open up (with the clinician's assistance) and disclose more information during the consultation. It is important to ask open-ended questions and avoid questions with simple yes or no responses. For example, when enquiring about the characteristics of a patient's back pain, don't ask, "Does the pain worsen when you bend down?" Instead, say, "Tell me, what are some of the activities which this pain restricts you from participating in?" The latter question elicits a more elaborate verbal response, in addition to identifying the different movements that exacerbate the patient's pain. Some dependent patients may also be introverted and would not divulge certain narrative information unless the question is posed in a particular way that encourages them to open up and be part of the dialogue.

In my past experiences, I've realized that picking a topic of interest for both the patient and me has been successful in getting the dependent patient to speak more during the clinical visit. The more the patient talks about a topic of interest, the less reserved the patient becomes. To encourage the patient to feel at ease in my presence, I will ask such questions as "So where are you from?" or "What line of work do you do?" If the patient is a parent, I may ask, "How old are your kids?" For the older patients who may be retired, I ask, "So what are your hobbies during these retirement years?" By asking these questions, I am not only forming a bond with my patients but I am also getting to know more about them. I obtain information that will ultimately assist me in making more efficient medical decisions. My general rule is to engage the patient in approximately five minutes of conversation on any topic of interest. This encourages the patient to become less reserved and more forthcoming with medical history. Once I notice that the patient is speaking freely and is less reserved, I then approach the issue of the reason for clinical visit. It works!

Trust between a clinician and a dependent patient is strengthened when the patient gets a sense that the clinician is not only interested in knowing what ails the patient but also wants to know who the patient is as an individual. It is truly amazing how much a clinician can accomplish during an initial visit with a new patient by investing a little time in a conversation with a patient, especially if the patient is new to the clinic. Investing about five minutes to get to know more about a patient is not a lot of time, given the great reward of a productive clinician-patient relationship.

CHAPTER EIGHT

The Skeptical Patient

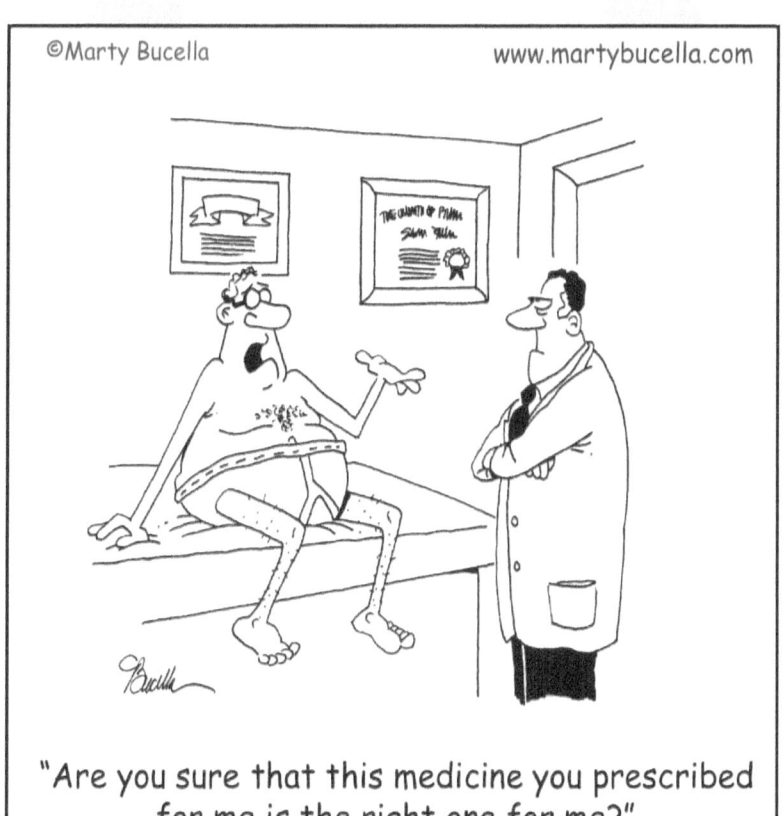

Nonye Tochi Aghanya, MSc, RN, FNP-C

Clinicians who have been in practice for many years may not routinely have encounters with the skeptical patient. However, new clinicians may come across the skeptical patient on a more regular basis. This is the patient who, at first contact, has a tendency to equate the clinician's clinical knowledge base with either the clinician's physical appearance, age, gender, or even race or nationality. I know that this may be a topic that does not frequently come up for discussion in the health care setting, but permit me to mention that it is very necessary to discuss it, because it is a contributory factor that plays a major role in communication development or breakdown between the patient and the clinician.

I remember an incident that took place sometime in 2002 during my practice in a subacute facility in the Bronx. I was an independent nurse practitioner and was occasionally assigned to that facility to manage patients' chronic ailments. I also assessed and provided treatment for acute illnesses. On this particular Monday morning, I was asked by a registered nurse to consult with one of the patients who had a low-grade fever for three days. I will refer to this patient as "Mrs. M." She was a fifty-four-year-old alert and self-sufficient patient who was admitted to the facility for rehabilitation services following a motor vehicle accident. She had made remarkable improvement since admission and did not require the nurse's assistance in performing activities of daily living. She was categorized as a self-treat patient. Patients in this category were admitted on a short course to the facility to receive respiratory therapy, physical therapy, or occupational therapy services. These patients were allowed to keep their medications in their own possession and self-administer per the clinician's instructions. They were very cognitively intact and aware of their environment, and they were active participants in their treatment plans and eventual discharges post-therapy. As their medical condition improved and they recovered from their injuries, self-treat patients were granted the privilege to temporarily leave the facility with use of an admittance pass for a few hours each day for personal errands.

Mrs. M was a self-treat patient. On this Monday morning, I was reminded by the nurse that Mrs. M had similar complaints on both Saturday and Sunday and was already seen twice by the clinician on call during the weekend. The nurse also mentioned to me that the on-call clinician prescribed some antibiotics for Mrs. M's symptoms. I thanked the nurse for the clinical update and smiled to myself as I walked down the long hallway that led to Mrs. M's room.

As I walked into her room, she sat at the edge of her bed, looked up at me with a puzzled facial expression, and said, "Oh, no—not another young one!" This statement caught me off guard, but I immediately started laughing. She appeared a bit perplexed and watched me for a while, and when she observed that I was not going to become offended, she laughed too.

When she laughed with me, I knew at this point that she had let her guard down a bit. And so, with an expression of amusement on my face, I said to her, "What do you mean? Do you think that I'm too young to treat you? Well, don't you worry. I'm sure I'll help you change your mind by the end of my visit with you." By verbalizing such a statement with a sense of humor and confidence, clinicians can improve the chances of achieving success in establishing an initial breakthrough with the skeptical patient. When a clinician is faced with such a patient skepticism on initial contact, it is vital that she refrain from displaying emotions that could be interpreted as being offended by skeptical remarks. This is because the skeptical patient watches the clinician's reactions very closely.

For this type of patient, initial trust must be established prior to implementing the next steps of consultation (history taking and physical exam). The clinician bears the burden of correcting any false misconceptions the patient may present with, and to date I've noticed that humor has remained the most effective approach for achieving a communication breakthrough with the skeptical patient. It is the first step of what I've termed the three steps of getting through to the skeptical patient.

Mrs. M told me that she was examined twice by another clinician, who recommended some antibiotics for an ear infection. She quickly quipped, "But my ear don't hurt and that doctor is young, so I don't think she knows what she is doing!" This is a typical case of patient skepticism.

I realized at that point that it was my responsibility to allay her fears, because she was now also applying such false perceptions she had about the previous "young" clinician to me. Unfortunately, patient perceptions (real or imagined) of the clinician sometimes play a big role in their level of compliance with the clinician's recommended medical plan of care. These perceptions may prevent the patient from fully implementing suggested clinical plans—or in worse cases, ignoring the plan entirely. In many cases, patients may not be eager to disclose their false perceptions, but once a clinician uses humor to initially engage the patient in a conversation, there is a natural instinct that most patients either directly or indirectly disclose their skepticisms to the clinician. This is because when a clinician encourages a patient to laugh, the patient feels more at ease and reveals his or her *true self,* which then encourages him or her to verbalize any lurking complaints, reservations, and false perceptions. Once Mrs. M felt at ease with my presence, in not so many words, she revealed to me that she did not trust the other clinician's medical judgment because of her youthful appearance. She insinuated that the clinician probably did not have enough medical experience to diagnose her correctly, so she stopped taking her antibiotics after the first dose.

Even though Mrs. M was forthright with me about her reservations, I knew that establishing complete trust was still an uphill battle because I was still "another young doctor," in her opinion. I reexamined Mrs. M and was not surprised to assess a left middle ear infection, which was already noted on her medical record by the previous clinician. Then I implemented the next step of trust establishment. For this step, the clinician needs to provide the patient with a brief medical background about the diagnosis (without unnecessary use of medical jargons). Mrs. M's report indicated she had an upper respiratory viral cold about six days prior to her initial complaint of a low-grade fever. I informed her that the URI (head cold) she'd had a few days ago could have contributed to her middle ear infection, because some fluid was trapped in the middle ear and caused it to become infected. I further informed her that some people with ear infections may not initially experience any distinct ear pain and that it could manifest as a variety of other symptoms such as dizziness, headache, fatigue, fever, tender lymph nodes, or body aches. Providing Mrs. M with this information took me no more than three minutes, and it achieved an immediate, overwhelmingly positive effect in trust development.

The final step was to encourage Mrs. M to take her antibiotics and complete it as recommended by the previous clinician. She assured me that she would do so, as she quickly proceeded to take a dose in my presence. She was pleased with the consultation, thanked me immensely, and asked me if I could become her regular doctor once she was discharged to the community. I was unable to do so because I did not have a private practice at that time. Although it initially appeared as though Mrs. M's reservation was about the probability of a misdiagnosed infection, it really was not about that concern at all. Mrs. M's actions revealed her desire for a clinician who would assist her in overcoming her skepticism about young doctors being medically unqualified to care for her, as well as a clinician who would also help her to develop a trusting relationship.

In summary, when a clinician encounters a skeptical patient, the overall goal should be to perceive and address the patient's reservations in a nonthreatening manner, and to simultaneously reveal your true identity to the patient as the knowledgeable, caring, and confident clinician that you believe you are. Such is your true identity, regardless of the perceptions (real or imagined) of the skeptical patient.

Nonye Tochi Aghanya, MSc, RN, FNP-C

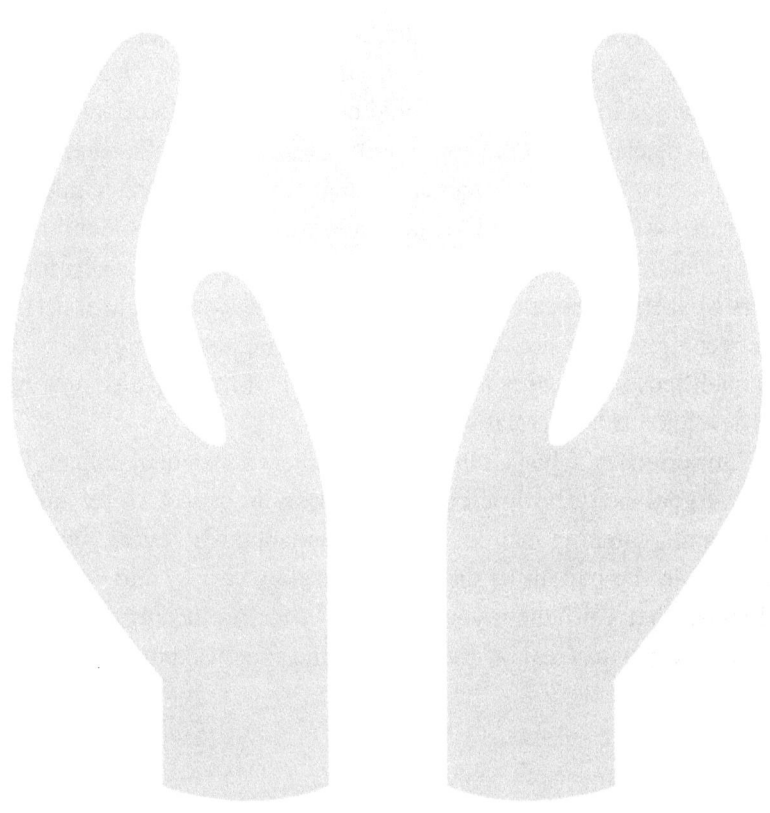

CHAPTER NINE

The Suspicious Patient

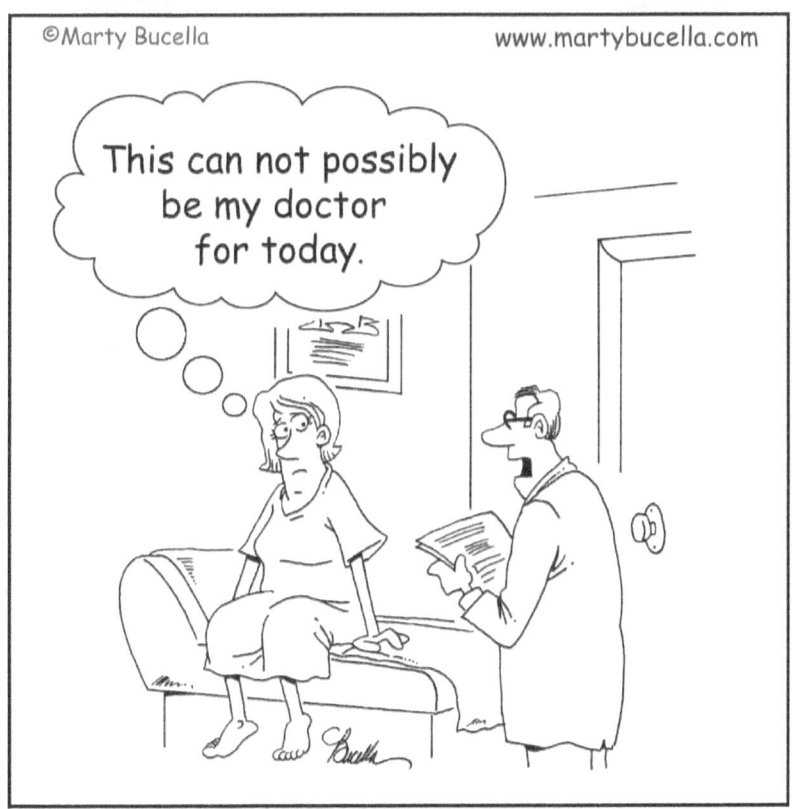

I wondered whether I should dedicate an entire chapter to describing the suspicious patient, because this patient's traits and characteristics are somewhat similar to those of the skeptical patient. I then realized that despite the similarities between both patients, in order to gain the trust of the suspicious patient, the clinician would need to implement a different approach. The suspicious patient is one with whom many new clinicians would also probably have an encounter during the early years of practice.

Many years ago, in my second year of practice, I walked into an exam room for a consultation with a sixty-eight-year-old male patient, whom I'll refer to as "Mr. O." He was reading a newspaper as I walked in. He raised his head for a moment, took a quick glance at me, and resumed reading his paper. "Good morning, Mr. O," I said. "I am Ms. Aghanya, your nurse practitioner for today."

His eyes darted upward, but his head didn't move. "Who are you again?" he asked. "I'm Ms. Aghanya, your nurse practitioner for today," I repeated. He then looked up at me and stated, "So you are the doctor? I was expecting someone a bit older."

Rather than feel offended, I felt quite flattered and took that as a compliment on my youthful appearance. Unfortunately, I don't get many such statements these days, since I can't say that I've maintained that youthful look over the years.

As a new clinician, your initial contact with the suspicious patient may create a moment of self-doubt, confusion, or intimidation. The first point to remember is to not panic or get offended. In addition, please do not ignore the patient's concern. The key to a successful dialogue is to acknowledge the patient's concern while attempting to establish a tone for respectful, engaging, and truthful conversation with the patient. I have always achieved this by briefly describing to the patient the steps I've taken in the previous years to establish and build my medical knowledge base and expertise. I share with the patient some information about my past education and previous work experiences in a relatable manner and a confident tone. This is usually the initial step for effective consultation with the suspicious patient.

The next step in establishing trust development occurs during the assessment and physical examination process. The goal is to allay the fears and diminish the patient's suspicions. I have found that speaking out loud my clinical-assessment findings for the patient to hear is a simple technique that helps reduce the suspicious patient's anxiety. For example, while auscultating lung sounds, as the patient inhales and exhales, I say, "Excellent. Breath sounds are clear." While assessing the ears with the otoscope, based on my findings, I would say, "Ear looks great; there is no redness. A little bit of fluid in the middle ear, but this is not unusual during this time of allergy season." For heart auscultation, I say, "Heartbeat is strong and steady, with a range that is within normal range." If I come across abnormal findings during the exam, I also verbalize that for the patient. Mr. O had some hard wax in the ear canal, and I stated to him, "Oh, I see some dark brown wax in your left ear, but it does not seem to have completely blocked your ear canal. As it accumulates, this may sometimes cause hearing difficulty or even dizziness. I will recommend some wax softeners at the end of the visit for you to apply and soften the wax." Generally, this process of verbalizing clinical findings to the patient continues until the completion of the physical exam. For the suspicious patient, as much as I'm able to, I explain the scientific process behind my medical decisions before proceeding to give my medical recommendations based on the scientific evidence.

It is vital for clinicians (especially new clinicians) to know that although the technique of disclosing your clinical findings to patients may seem a daunting task that initially requires much effort for you to implement, this habit helps to improve your confidence in clinical practice as you observe a patient who was initially suspicious of your clinical skills gradually make a reversal and trust your medical decisions. As you get to know more about your patient and as your confidence level with the physical exam process improves, the suspicious patient becomes more trusting of your clinical judgments. Follow-up consultation visits with the patient will become easier to perform. This was definitely the case with Mr. O, who later made a request with the scheduling staff to schedule his subsequent medical appointments with me.

CHAPTER TEN

The Talkative Patient

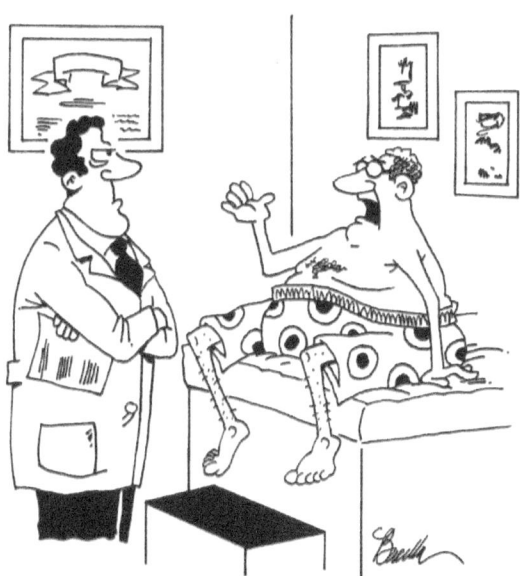

As a busy clinician, have you ever come across a patient who you actually wished would stop talking for just a second? I sure have met a few talkative patients in my years of medical practice. This is the patient who may ramble on and on, in an attempt to provide the clinician with a history during the clinical visit. Sometimes, the contents of the patient's history may be quite relevant to the consultation visit, but they may not be presented in a cohesive structure. There may be some flight of ideas that might make it quite challenging for the clinician to prioritize the patient's complaints and symptoms and determine a treatment plan for the most critical symptoms. This is because the talkative patient may have an underlying anxiety that makes it difficult for him to slow down, gather his thoughts, and then narrate the medical history in a precise manner. In this chapter, I will give illustrations of three scenarios of the talkative patient.

Scenario A. I consulted with "Mrs. W" a few years ago. She presented with complaints of an upper respiratory infection. Mrs. W had experienced some congestion for about three weeks and decided to visit the local clinic for assessment. She sat down opposite my desk, and I said, "Hello, Mrs. W, what can I do for you today?"

Mrs. W stated, "I had a head cold about three weeks ago, and I took some over-the-counter cough medicines. Although it kind of helped me a bit, I was still coughing so much at nighttime and noticed last night that I may be wheezing a bit. I was up all night because you know, it gets so warm during this time of the year, and it is so hard to fall asleep when the weather is really warm. When it gets so warm, my skin also gets very dry and begins to itch badly. I sat up in my bed all night and coughed a lot, and it seemed like I felt a little bit of chest pain. And yes, now I remember, my ears were also hurting, and right now my heart is beating really fast because I didn't get much sleep. I'm not sure if all these have affected my eyes because it seems like my right eye is suddenly oozing stuff from it." Quite a mouthful, right? Well, listening to all that information in that form made my head spin, but I remembered that the goal of communicating with such patient is to typically give the patient some time to verbalize her immediate concerns and then gradually assist her to concentrate, identify, and prioritize more critical symptoms. My approach in this scenario was to allow Mrs. W some time to verbalize all her concerns without much interruption. (Most narrative reports from the talkative patient typically last about two to three minutes, because as much as the patients enjoy talking, they usually run out of things to say within that frame of time before looking to the clinician to fix every problem they've just stated in the narrative report.) Once I realized that Mrs. W had completed verbalizing her complaints, I repeated to her what I believe I heard her say beginning with the most clinically relevant symptoms, in order to rule out any acute cardiac or respiratory-related ailments. Then I gradually expanded the conversation.

With a gentle but firm tone, I responded to Mrs. W. "Please correct me if I'm wrong, but I believe I heard you say that your chest was hurting at some point last night. Was that while you were coughing? Does it hurt when you take a deep breath? Or is it a chest pain that you've experienced throughout the night? Is your chest hurting as you sit here in the clinic right now?" Mrs. W replied that she did not experience any chest pains at rest, with exertion, or with deep inspiration; she experienced chest and side muscle pains only during moments of active coughing. Once I established by history that there were likely no acute cardiac or respiratory complaints that demanded immediate medical interventions, I was now able to gradually review the rest of Mrs. W's history with her. I gently said, "I also heard you say that you experienced some earache and drainage from your eyes." Mrs. W seemed more comfortable and attentive at this point, and she was glad to provide me with answers to all subsequent questions that I asked her. She also exhibited less flight of ideas as the visit progressed. It turned out that Mrs. W had acute bronchitis with an ear infection, and I treated her with antibiotics and cough expectorants. She made a complete recovery.

Scenario B. A second scenario of a talkative patient is one who presents to the consultation and, because of underlying anxiety about the visit, quickly wants to break the ice by being overly talkative as a means to reduce any perceived tensions in the clinic. On many occasions, I've found that these tensions do not really exist but are only perceived or imagined by the patient. Once seated, such a patient immediately starts the visit by talking about personal and private life events with the hope that this will help him break the ice and experience a pleasant visit with the clinician. Some patients do not recognize that dwelling on a nonclinical subject during the history-taking process becomes a distraction for the clinician and a deterrent to building a meaningful relationship. I will refer to the patient in this scenario as "Mr. T." Early on a cold November morning, Mr. T presented to the local clinic in his neighborhood with complaints of congestion. While narrating the medical history to the clinician, he stated, "I was on a cruise last week and developed this cough and congestion after I returned two day ago. Wow, what a cruise it was! Have you ever been on the Norwegian cruise line? That cruise has the best cuisine and entertainment I've experienced in a long time."

This patient's approach of giving a medical history to the clinician may initially seem friendly and inviting to the new clinician but I have found it to be very counterproductive because it quickly diverts attention from the main reason for clinical visit to more trivial or nonclinical issues. Moreover, if the clinician becomes intrigued and distracted by the patient's conversations, less emphasis is placed on the relevant clinical reason for the visit. This could result in a substandard medical decision-making process. In the scenario with Mr. T, the goal was to redirect the patient to the main clinical reason for his visit without seemingly dismissing his conversation points. One way that I succeeded in doing this was to conduct the patient's history and physical exam without engaging in any in-depth conversation with the patient at first. I would give simple yes or no responses and deliberately would not engage the patient in long conversations. However, as the physical exam progressed, I would gradually reintroduce the patient's conversation points with findings of the physical exam, as applicable. Let me give you an example.

With Mr. T's scenario, it was unwise to disclose to the talkative

Tips for Effective Communication: A Vital Tool for Trust Development

patient such information that created an opportunity for the patient to further divert from the main clinical complaint. In response to his question, I smiled at Mr. T and said, "No, Mr. T, I have never been on a Norwegian cruise line. It sure sounds like fun, but let's focus on those symptoms you've experienced since you returned from your cruise. It could be possible that the cruise cabins were cooler than normal, and you were exposed to cold drafts in the cabin which is why you developed cold symptoms. What other symptoms do you experience at this time?" This refocuses conversation to the clinical history, and after obtaining the history, I began the physical exam. While performing Mr. T's physical exam, I gradually made reference to some of his earlier conversation points about the cruise line. His blood pressure was within normal limits, and I said, "Your blood pressure is really great today. It seems like that cruise was relaxing, as you mentioned, and the experience has helped improve your blood pressure." Assuming Mr. T was a diabetic, following my review of his weight and blood glucose levels, I noticed no weight fluctuations or blood sugar level abnormalities. I said, "It seems like you've done well to maintain a steady weight and normal blood sugar levels in the past few months. This is quite an accomplishment, especially with all the great food choices you mentioned were available on your recent cruise. I'm glad you're making the right choices with regards to your health."

This is a unique approach that places more emphasis on clinical visit reports without dismissing the patient's attempts to engage the clinician in a friendly conversation. It helps achieve a productive clinician-patient relationship.

Scenario C. In the third scenario, a patient may come to the clinic, and rather than provide information about the clinical reason for the visit, she would speak incessantly about the weather or traffic patterns, or parking restriction issues that she encountered on the way to the clinic visit. I have come across this scenario on numerous occasions, and I typically listen briefly and acknowledge the patient's concern with the following response. "Wow, I'm sorry to hear you had such a bad experience trying to get here today. Hopefully, your blood pressure is not affected by the experience.

We should probably hold off on checking your blood pressure till later in the visit. I'm glad you finally made it in. So what brings you to the clinic today?" Clinicians should make every effort to never dismiss a patient's complaints, no matter how trivial it may initially seem to the clinician. It is important to offer some form of acknowledgment before redirecting the course of the visit to the patient's chief complaint. It goes a long way toward trust development between the patient and the clinician.

These are just a few of the many scenarios I've encountered over my years of practice. Patients in these three scenarios represent so many patients that are out there in our hospitals, clinics, and emergency rooms, and they simply wish to have a positive experience with their clinicians. I am neither a psychiatrist nor a psychologist, but at some point in my life, I was also a patient who experienced that common fear and anxiety that patients have as they communicate with their clinicians. As a clinician, I have also communicated with various patients over the course of many years. Both roles have helped me to develop a heartfelt belief that all human beings have a deep-rooted need to be heard, acknowledged, and appreciated. In different clinical situations, the clinician, as a professional figure bears the responsibility to listen to the patient and detect when and how to impose limits on some patient's unrealistic expectations while promoting an atmosphere that encourages the patient to engage freely in uninhibited and honest communication.

CHAPTER ELEVEN

The Dr. Moms and Dr. Dads

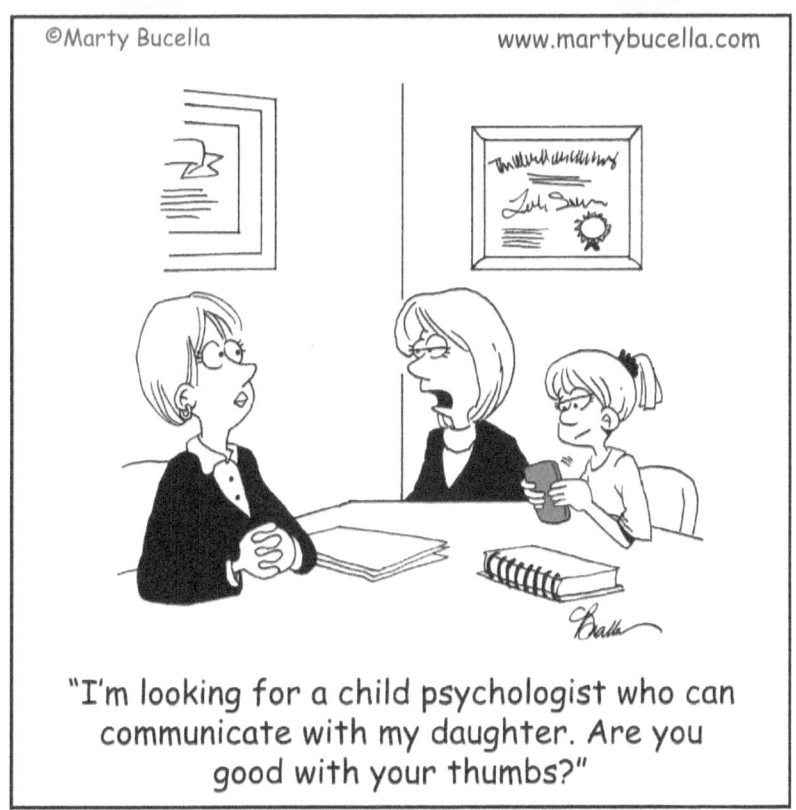

As a clinician, I have made it a priority to never dispute or underestimate any clinical input from the parents of a pediatric patient. Parents care deeply for their children, and sometimes such caring attitude can manifest as an excessive attempt to make things right. For many clinicians, there will come a time when a parent may seem a bit overly enthusiastic about his or her contribution to the clinical visit. Some parents may actually develop the impression that given their in-depth knowledge of their children's traits, characteristics, and behavior patterns, they reserve the right to inform the clinician of what to do and what medications should be prescribed for their children.

Such parents have the tendency to arrive at a clinic visit with formed opinions and beliefs regarding the etiology and treatment plans for the child's ailments. The parents may say, "I know the medicine my child needs, because that's what my child took in the past that made him feel better." There is some truth to such statements because many pediatric ailments that are encountered in the outpatient medical clinics are common ailments (e.g., ear infections, rash, strep infections, viral infections), and these respond to very specific treatment plans. However, clinicians should bear in mind that encouraging this communication pattern with the overbearing parent would limit room for open conversations and in-depth communication that is necessary for exploring the etiology of other uncommon complaints that the child may present with at subsequent visits. Also, by not adequately addressing or correcting such parental impressions, a new clinician promotes the risk of becoming intimidated when the sick child presents for a future visit with an uncommon ailment.

My first few months of clinical practice were in an outpatient pediatric clinic in Paterson, New Jersey. As a new clinician, I knew that I needed to improve my confidence in clinical practice, but the encounters I had with the overly enthusiastic parents made it a bit difficult to improve on my clinical confidence. I noticed at some point that I was beginning to rely heavily on the parental input in order to arrive at a medical decision, based solely on the parents' observations or what they had studied in some literature about the child's symptoms. It was difficult to communicate effectively because the parents often told me what the child's symptoms were, what they felt was wrong with the child and what medication the child needed because "this medicine worked fine in the past for my child." As I permitted this pattern of communication to continue, I began to get the sense that my role in the consultation was simply to use my prescriptive privileges to prescribe the medication suggested by the parents, because the parents did not have the prescriptive authority to do so.

At this point, I had to stop and ask myself, "What am I missing, and how can I improve my interactions with these parents?" It took me a few more months to finally figure it out. I worked hard to establish a pattern of communication that has benefited both me and the parents of my pediatric patients. Please don't get me wrong: as a clinician, I appreciate and consider every parent's concerns and contributions to each clinical visit as vital information. But I will frankly mention that I've come across some Dr. Moms and Dr. Dads whose perspectives can be so intrusive that it becomes a deterrent to building an honest, trusting relationship. There are instances when a clinician encounters a parent whose expectations, style of communication, and mannerisms could be viewed as overbearing. This can have a negative impact on effective history taking for the clinician. Sometimes, such scenarios could become a bit intimidating for a new clinician, creating an atmosphere for a new clinician to doubt his or her clinical skills during the decision-making process.

When a clinician is faced with such a situation, it is vital that she take a step back, reanalyze the current communication pattern, and emerge with ways to improve such interaction with the child's parents. The parental role during the clinical visit is invaluable, and the parents' contribution is priceless in obtaining a targeted history and establishing an accurate medical diagnosis and treatment plan for the sick child. However, if a clear distinction is not established with an overbearing parent, especially during the initial clinical visits, the parents could constantly arrive at a premature medical conclusion based on information obtained from various sources (reliable and unreliable). A new clinician can become easily intimidated and can depend heavily (or solely) on the clinical suggestions by a Dr. Mom or Dr. Dad, which leads to a counterproductive parent-clinician interaction.

This chapter highlights some of the common characteristics of a Dr. Mom or Dr. Dad. It provides illustrations and insights to the best approach that I've utilized over the course of many years, ensuring that although I don't dismiss a parent's contributions to the clinical visit; I also make every effort, in a nonthreatening manner, to establish my primary role to the parent as that of the child's clinician. The important point to remember as a clinician is that more times than not, parents can identify the progression of their children's symptoms and illness. The information they provide to the clinician is valuable and should never be discredited, regardless of how it is relayed. The goal for the new clinician is to have a positive visit encounter without undermining parental contributions, while emphasizing your role and maintaining the responsibility as the clinician to direct the flow of the visit and implement the most appropriate medical plan of care.

The following three scenarios show in detail some successful approaches to use when interacting with a Dr. Mom or Dr. Dad. These approaches have enabled me to develop and maintain a trusting relationship with the parents of my pediatric patients.

Scenario A. I once had a clinic visit encounter with an eleven-year-old boy and his mother. I'll refer to the parent as "Mrs. R." The patient presented with a complaint of lingering sore throat for two days. As I obtained more information about the chief complaint, I spoke to the patient and his mother about the history of symptoms. With a warm smile and in a gentle tone, I asked the boy, "Did you have a stuffy nose and congestion before you first felt that your throat was sore?"

Before the child had a chance to respond to my question, the parent immediately stated, "I really believe that this is strep, because this is how he usually feels when he gets strep. You should do a strep test now, and maybe send a culture to the lab too." My initial reaction was a bit of shock as I observed the eleven-year-old boy, who was getting ready to respond to my question before the mother quipped in. He suddenly appeared embarrassed, shut down, and stopped making any attempt to respond to my question.

Rather than feel upset or insulted by the parent's attempt to tell me how to practice, I said, "You know what? You are absolutely right, Mrs. R, and it's definitely a good idea to send out a throat sample for a confirmatory strep DNA test for all rapid strep tests with negative results. However, I will go ahead and obtain the rest of the history so that I'll know whether a strep test is medically needed. Sometimes, some viral cold symptoms can present with sore throat because of postnasal drip, which can easily be mistaken for a strep throat infection." I obtained the rest of the history and proceeded to examine the eleven-year-old patient.

Over the years of practice, I've observed that keeping such enthusiastic parents informed of your clinical findings with each step of the medical exam process helps reduce parental anxiety (which ultimately reduces the child's anxiety). This is because most pediatric patients look to their parents to make them feel comfortable during clinical visits, and they inherently take on their parents' emotions as they observe the parents' reactions to the clinician during the visit. I then said to the mother, "He doesn't have a fever, and by the looks of his throat, I really don't see an obvious appearance of strep which is typically a beefy red patch or red spots. I also don't see any brown or white patches, and his tonsils are not swollen. However, his right lymph node is slightly enlarged, and his right middle ear is a bit reddened with some clear fluid, which is sometimes seen following a viral head cold. It does not always mean that the ear is infected. In many occasions, the constant dripping of postnasal fluid to the throat causes soreness of throat. Sometimes, children do not present with the classic symptoms of strep, and I remember you mentioned that your son had similar symptoms in the past when he was diagnosed with strep throat. Let us perform a rapid strep test and send an overnight sample to the lab so that we don't miss anything."

Have you noticed what I've accomplished with this pattern of communication? I expanded on the parent's immediate concern that was disclosed at the onset, and I acknowledged the parent's recommendation. While I spoke, I also took the time to reestablishing my role as the child's clinician by bringing to the parent's attention other simple differential diagnosis and the rationale for my medical judgments. It is vital to accomplish this without the use of medical jargon, expand on the parent's presumed diagnosis for the child—and to do so while keeping the parent informed of all simple clinical findings. Such enthusiastic parents tend to appreciate this approach, which helps foster a trusting and respectful parent-clinician relationship.

Scenario B. A mother (whom I'll refer to as Mrs. P) came to the clinic with her six-year-old son, who complained of sore throat for three days. While I was obtaining a medical history regarding the pain characteristics and fever status, Mrs. P interrupted me midsentence, and with steady eye contact very confidently stated, "Well, my child got the flu shot last month, so this cannot possibly be a throat infection because I know the flu shot lowers the chances of these kinds of infections." She sounded so confident, and if it had been in my early years of practice as a brand-new clinician, I probably would have felt a bit intimidated and may not have responded or corrected Mrs. P's partially false clinical assumptions.

Many times during a visit, new clinicians are eager to establish a good relationship with the parents of sick children, and they will more likely respond or interact with parents in such ways that will limit disagreements. In this scenario, a new clinician may likely ignore Mrs. P's statement, proceed with the rest of history taking, conduct a physical exam, probably diagnose the child with a bacteria or viral upper respiratory infection, and prescribe the appropriate treatment plan at the end of the visit. Clinicians (especially new clinicians) may opt for such an approach for various reasons to avoid addressing the parent's false clinical assumptions because they may think, *"I do not wish to make parents feel uncomfortable, ruffle any feathers, or create unnecessary tension during the visit."* They want the parent to feel satisfied with the visit.

If a clinician chooses to not address or correct Mrs. P's false assumptions, it is important to note that a complete clinical visit could still be achieved because the child's clinical complaints would be addressed in a tension- free atmosphere. However, by not addressing Mrs. P, the parent retains this false clinical assumption, and she will most likely continue to apply it during subsequent visits. This creates a recipe for poor communication and deters the development of a meaningful parent-clinician relationship.

My approach to Mrs. P's comment was to gently but firmly correct her as I said to her, "You are somewhat correct that the flu shot reduces the chances of getting the flu, Mrs. P. But please know that there are other organisms that can cause infections, such as bacterial, yeast, or fungal infections. The symptoms of viral, bacterial, or even fungal infections are sometimes similar on initial appearance, so it is great that you brought in your child to be examined today, so that we can examine him and run some tests to determine what kind of infection he has."

This statement has achieved three major purposes.

1.) It acknowledged the parental input and commended the parental diagnosis while revealing its partial correctness.

2.) Without use of medical jargon, it provided a simple explanation regarding other clinical possibilities without totally dismissing parental input.

3.) It further extended the dialogue to inform the parent of the possibility for further lab tests as appropriate.

Scenario C. A father (whom I'll refer to as Mr. D) came to the clinic with his nine-year-old son, who complained of ear pressure for five days. During history assessment, Mr. D said, "I really believe my child's ears are blocked with wax, because I have a history of wax and I read somewhere that it is hereditary. I have been putting earwax drops in his ears for the past three days, but he is still complaining of pressure."

At this point, all new clinicians should remember the general rule: reaffirm what is true about the parent's statement and correct any false clinical assumptions while disclosing other clinical possibilities that may be pertinent to the patient's complaints. My response to Mr. D was, "You are right about the possibility of ear pressure signifying wax buildup, especially given the fact that there is a family history. But please know that ear pressure can also be experienced with many other medical conditions such as outer or middle ear infections. For the future, know that it's not usually a good idea to instill any drops without having the ears first examined. But it's great you brought in your child so that we can determine the possible cause of his ear pressure."

This reaffirmed Mr. D's concerns, corrected any misconceptions, and commended his attempt to seek clinical consultation. Following the exam, it was noted that the child had an infection in both middle ears with no wax accumulation. Antibiotics were prescribed and the parent was advised to stop applying the wax-softening drops. Mr. D was appreciative and happy that he didn't need to continue applying drops that his son did not need.

In order for effective communication to be accomplished, the patterns of the three scenarios can be duplicated and applied in other instances once a parent is identified as a Dr. Mom or Dr. Dad. To achieve success, the clinician must be knowledgeable about the clinical subject and strive to gently and confidently relay that knowledge without appearing intimidating or dismissive. Never underestimate the power of your clinical knowledge and skills. Never stop learning!

Another key to effective communication is a simple one: the clinician's manner of approach. If a parent seems tired, overwhelmed, or anxious, I recognize that the child's illness must be contributory to the parent's emotional state, and thus I'm not easily irritated. I've also made it a habit to address parents as Mom or Dad in the course of clinical conversations. To a parent who presents to the clinic with a four-year-old child named Alicia, I begin a history-taking process with, "Okay, Mom, what brings you in today with little Alicia? She seems tired and quite clingy to you, which I'm sure has made it a very exhausting day for you." Parents appreciate when clinicians acknowledge the impact that the child's illness may have on their lives. It is a simple step that opens the door for honest, effective communication between the clinician and the parent of a sick child. The following are common dos and don'ts for communication success with a Dr. Mom or Dr. Dad.

Common Don'ts

Once a clinician identifies an overly enthusiastic parent, especially at an initial visit:
- Do not panic
- Do not feel offended or angry
- Do not feel inadequate or incompetent
- Do not feel that the parent is undermining your clinical skills
- Do not feel that the parent is telling you what to do
- Do not feel that the parent does not trust your clinical judgment
- Do not feel rushed to come to a clinical decision
- Do not become dismissive of the parent's input

Rather, Practice These Common Dos

- Know that the overly enthusiastic parent cares for the sick child
- Be confident and know that your medical knowledge is instrumental in establishing trust with the parent
- Take time to explain disease process, other common differential diagnosis, and treatment options
- Maintain an atmosphere of confidence without appearing dismissive
- Always dress professionally
- Keep up your knowledge with continuous medical education; attend medical seminars
- *Never stop learning.* Knowledge shared with compassion is the key to establishing a meaningful clinician-parent-patient relationship.

Nonye Tochi Aghanya, MSc, RN, FNP-C

-

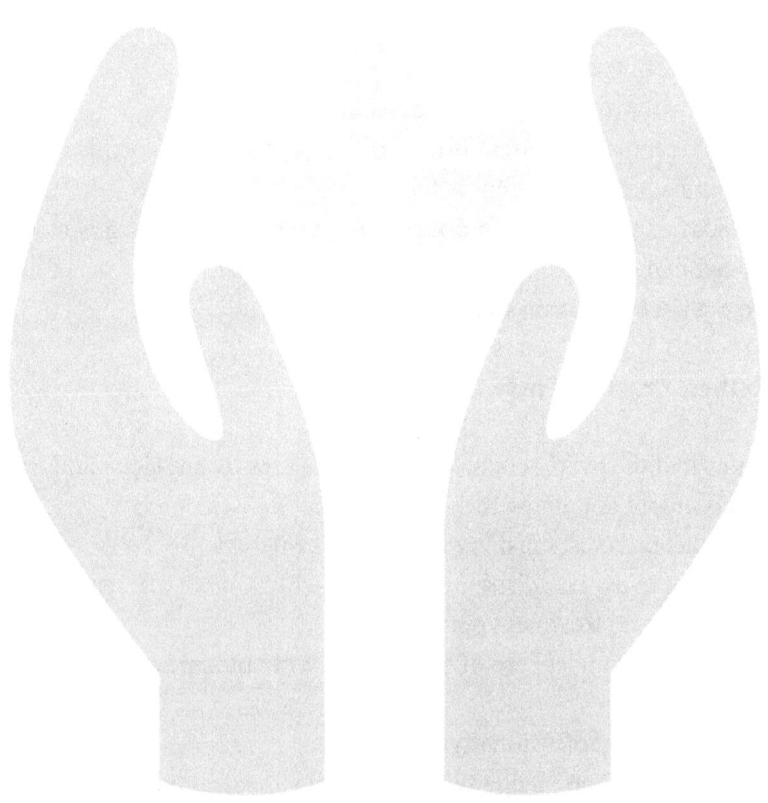

CHAPTER TWELVE
The Overwhelmed Patient

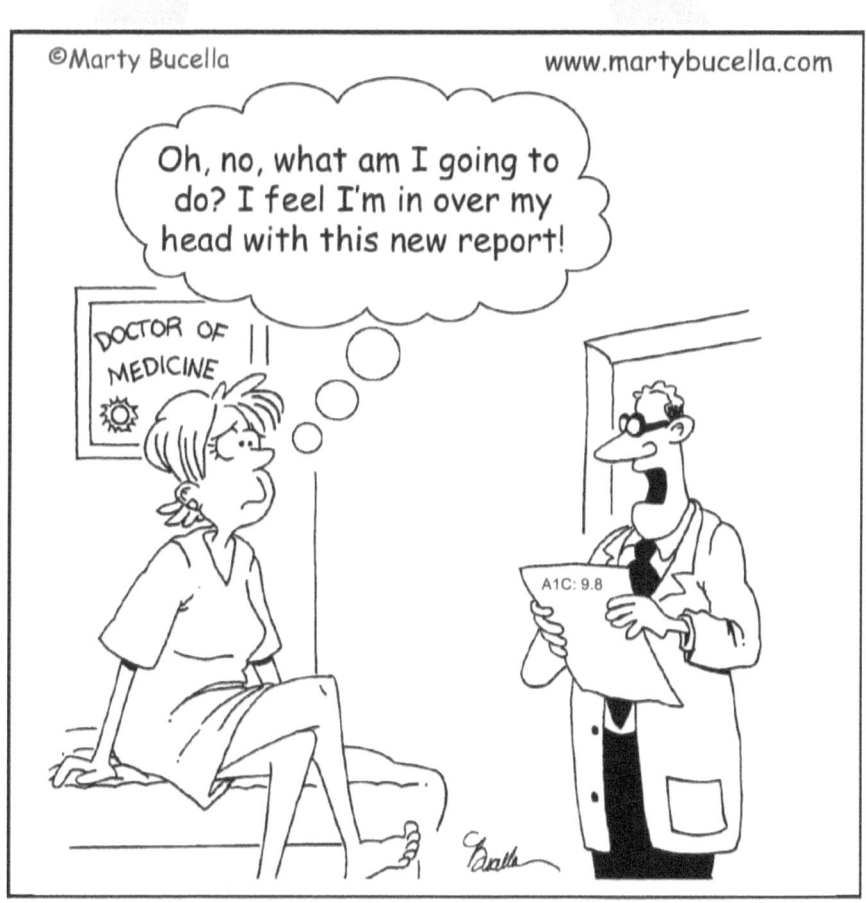

In this category, the clinician may be dealing with a patient who is newly diagnosed with a chronic ailment (e.g., diabetes). There is a comprehensive learning need for the newly diagnosed diabetic patient. With the demand for immediate change in lifestyle, diet, and exercise activities, the newly diagnosed diabetic patient will likely feel overwhelmed by these requirements, and the tons of educational information associated with the ailment. It is important to note that the overwhelmed patient is more likely to benefit from a teaching session that is presented in bits at a time. Patients take away nuggets each time they consult with the clinician. Only pertinent information should be shared at the initial visit; too much information should not be divulged because patients usually do not take away the entire piece at the first visit. A newly diagnosed diabetic patient may ask, "Do I need to do all these lifestyle and diet changes, and test my sugar levels every day?" The following are two kinds of clinical responses.

- **Statement A:** "Yes, you need to do so in order to maintain normal blood sugar levels, which will help to prevent organ damage in the future."
-
- **Statement B:** "It is important to change your current diet and lifestyle in order to improve your blood sugar levels, but you actually really do not need to make all these changes at once. How about focusing on just one or two changes and doing them well? Then, let's see where we go from there."

Note that although statement A is an accurate statement, its vague delivery structure would likely not help the patient feel any less overwhelmed. This is because statement A points toward a demand for an immediate modification of dietary and lifestyle changes that is not realistic. It scares the overwhelmed patient when these requirements are not met within a short period of time. Patients may feel beaten down, guilty, and scared to open up to the clinician, which further deters effective communication.

However, in a more realistic way, statement B informs the patient of the importance of diet and lifestyle modification. This delivery structure is less intimidating and offers the option for the patient to gradually prioritize what aspects of lifestyle changes should initially be focused on.

The goal of having a conversation with the overwhelmed patient is to involve the patient in the process of reaching a medical plan of care that would promote compliance without further overwhelming the patient. Most patients may feel anxious with the presumption that their current comfortable lifestyles will be suddenly altered by the clinician's suggestions. Many patients prefer to maintain control of the required dietary and lifestyle modifications. They would rather incorporate clinical suggestions and make adjustments based on their existing schedule, rather than completely altering their current lifestyles. Given that learning needs for effective diabetes management are quite complex, many clinicians opt to refer the newly diagnosed patient to a diabetes educator for a tailored teaching plan that is specific to the patient.

Clinician and patient expectations for the management of hypertension, another common chronic ailment, may also create overwhelming emotions for some patients. Most people with elevated blood pressure generally feel healthy and are asymptomatic, so they may not have a full grasp of the expectations for effective blood pressure management. Thus, conversations between clinician and patient regarding the complications of high blood pressure (e.g., kidney disease, heart attack, stroke, aneurysms) could further overwhelm the patient. If the clinician determines that a patient will need to take an oral hypertensive agent, it is more appropriate to use a conversational approach that will give the patient an opportunity to reflect on his current lifestyle and arrive at the most conducive plan that will promote compliance with the clinician's recommendations. For instance, let's examine these two statements by the clinician.

- **Statement A:** "I am going to prescribe [medication name] for you. This will help with your hypertension management, and this is the time of day you should be taking it (e.g., every morning at nine o'clock). How confident are you that you can take it this medication at that time of day every day?"

-
- **Statement B:** "I will also recommend that you keep track of your blood pressure levels. Various pharmacy locations have the self-monitoring electronic blood pressure devices installed in the stores. There is also the option of buying a self-monitoring BP device. Would you be able to take the time to go a pharmacy and check your blood pressure about three times a week? Or do you feel that purchasing a monitor and checking it at home would be easier?"

These statements provide the patient an opportunity to explore various options with the clinician regarding blood pressure management. Obtaining the patient's input during this process encourages self-directed behavioral changes for the patient. The clinician should also remember that patients may commonly feel intimidated as they struggle to come to terms with the fact that their existing lifestyle will be modified. It is common to find that during this period, some patients in their overwhelmed state feel hesitant to interrupt the clinician and ask questions about their medical plan of care. Thus, the clinician should always strive to implement a conversational approach of communication with the overwhelmed patient. For many years, I've used the following open invitation statement with my patients, and it has helped alleviate anxiety. "If what I'm saying does not make any sense to you at any point, please feel free to stop me so that we can clarify it together." Such a pattern of statement encourages interaction and is necessary in developing a productive relationship with the overwhelmed patient. Otherwise, following a consultation, the patient could leave with an impression that the clinician's views and instructions were imposed on him or her and this false impression will overwhelm the patient even further!

Tips for Effective Communication: A Vital Tool for Trust Development

CHAPTER THIRTEEN
The Impatient Patient

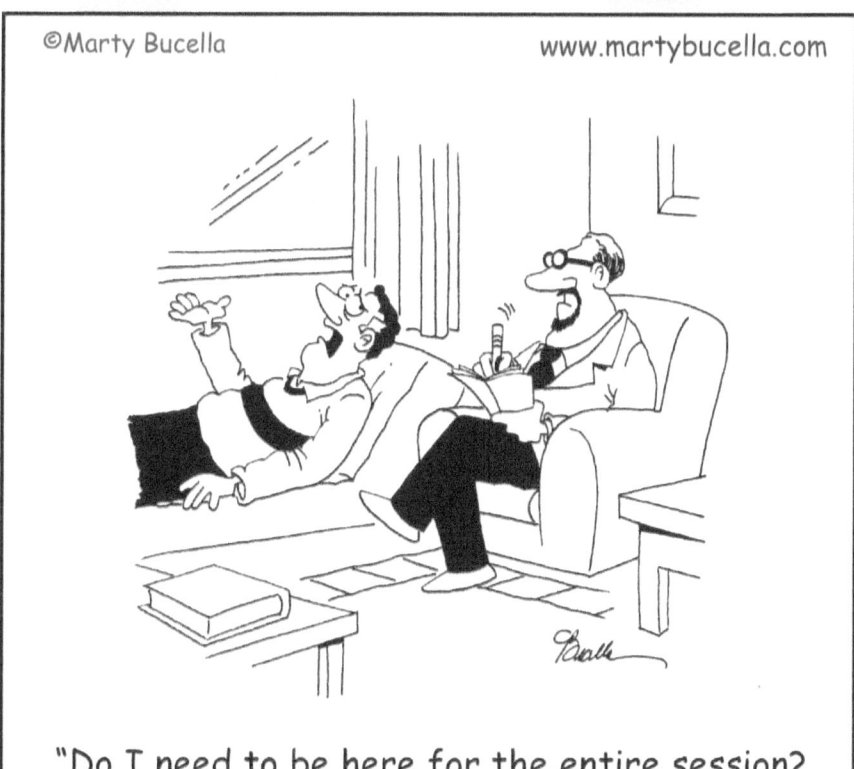

"Do I need to be here for the entire session? I really need to be somewhere else in the next 30 minutes."

Many clinicians with well-established relationships with their patients may not have frequent encounters with the impatient patient. However, a new patient's consultation with a clinician creates the most likely environment and opportunity for a patient to exhibit the characteristics of an impatient patient. In the various locations that clinicians consult with patients (hospital, outpatient primary care medical clinics, home care, subacute, and urgent care), more often than in any other clinical setting, the impatient patient is encountered in the urgent clinic or walk-in settings. This is the patient who always seems to be in a hurry during a consultation. Although difficult to imagine, there are patients that will nudge the clinician along during a visit. For example, a patient may intermittently glance at his or her watch, or occasionally stare at a wall clock during a consultation visit. In some rare instances, patients may make it crystal clear to the clinician that they are in a hurry.

Many years ago, during my early years in practice in New York, I had an experience with a patient who stated, "Could you please hurry up? I need to be in a meeting in thirty minutes." Sometimes patients may indicate that they need to catch a flight, pick up a kid, attend a meeting, or do some shopping. For a new clinician, this can become a distraction and if it's not addressed appropriately, it can become a deterrent to establishing a meaningful relationship. Any clinician who encounters an impatient patient must first realize that the patient's behavior discloses the fact that the clinician has not developed a meaningful relationship with the patient, and thus the clinician should set a goal to develop one. A patient who has a respectful and meaningful relationship with his or her clinician is rarely an impatient patient. As detailed in previous chapters of this book, regardless of a patient's characteristics and communication style during a visit, the burden of establishing a trusting and meaningful relationship eventually lies with the clinician. This patient typically displays a shorter attention span with limited listening skills during consultations. This could frustrate a new clinician and negatively impact the normal flow of communication. Generally, effective communication is vital to developing a meaningful relationship with all patients.

Once I observe such a patient during a clinical visit, I usually quickly inform the patient of my awareness of the patient's apparent haste and discomfort with the current pace of the consultation visit. I achieve this by gently stating, "I notice that you're frequently glancing at your watch, which makes it appear that you are in a hurry. Is there somewhere you need to be that is more important than this visit?" This approach opens up an opportunity for a dialogue with the patient. I have noticed that once I ask this question, many patients are usually quite surprised that I bothered to inquire about the reason for their impatience. In most scenarios, this patient reevaluates his or her actions and gradually refrains from the unreasonable demand to rush the clinician through the clinic visit. I then explain to the patient that a thorough history and physical examination is necessary so that we can make an accurate diagnosis and provide the most appropriate treatment plan. It is important that the clinician not ignore obvious indicators of an impatient patient. It ought to be addressed immediately, to encourage a more conducive and tension-free atmosphere for the remainder of the clinic visit.

There have been instances where patients may truly have an emergent situation that requires an early conclusion to the visit. The opportunity for an open dialogue initiated by the clinician will help determine this (e.g., a parent could be contacted by the child's school during consultation visit because of an emergency in school). In such a case, the visit is terminated, and the patient can reschedule his or her appointment in order to address the emergent situation. The clinician should refrain from rushing through a consultation visit in order to meet the demands of the impatient patient, because this encourages the patient to continue to act in such a manner for subsequent visits, which does not contribute to the development of a meaningful clinician-patient relationship.

Nonye Tochi Aghanya, MSc, RN, FNP-C

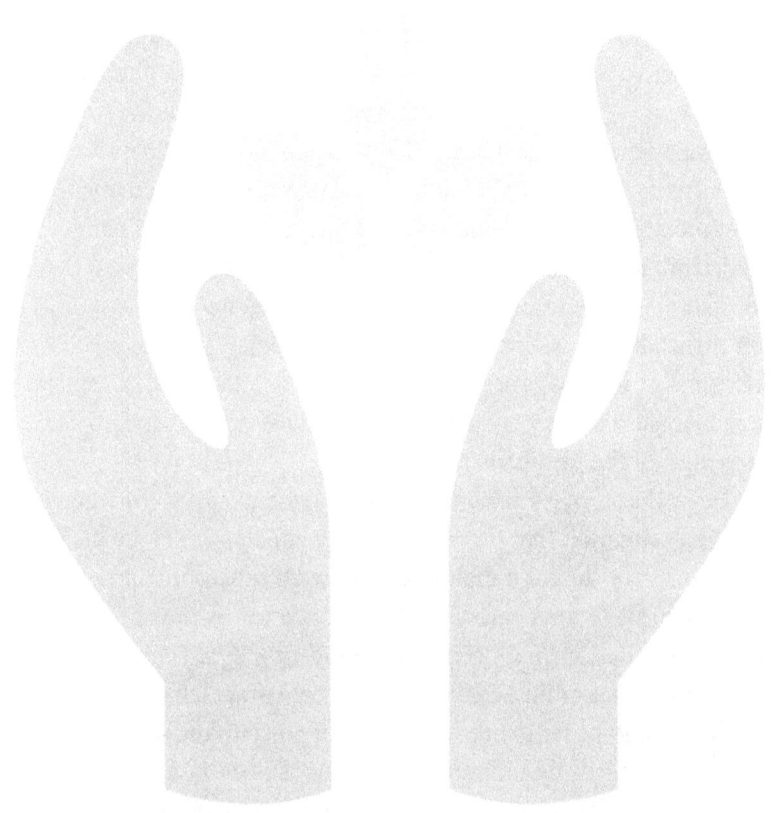

CHAPTER FOURTEEN

When the Patient Is a Health Care Provider

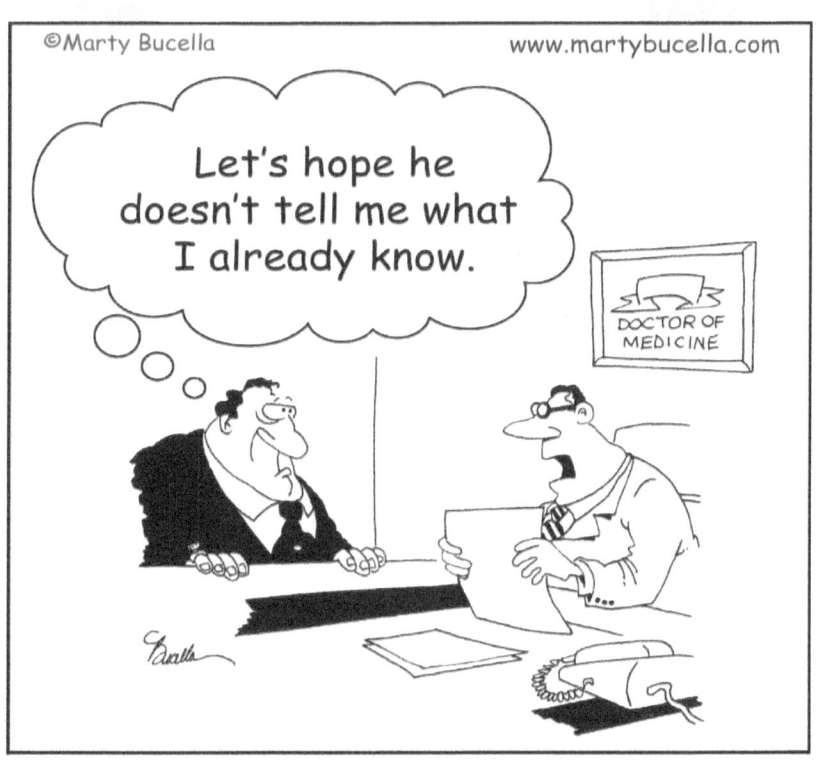

Occasionally, the treating clinician may have a patient who is a health care provider with limited (or sometimes extensive) knowledge of the health care system, disease process, and treatment options. For the new clinician, a realization that your patient is also a medical provider may initially seem a bit awkward as you reflect on what existing knowledge the patient may have about his or her medical condition. As a new clinician, I remember being quite anxious that I would "mess up the visit" and I was always so conscious of the patient's status as a health care provider that I either had a frozen or no personality during such visits! One thing I've realized over the years is that for a treating clinician to gain the trust of a patient who is also a medical provider, the treating clinician must maintain a sense of calm and confidence. It is quite common for a new clinician to experience a moment of self-doubt at the realization that a patient is also a health care provider.

Whenever I encounter this scenario, my initial goal remains the same: to implement a plan that will assist the patient in feeling at ease in my presence. When a patient tells me, "Oh, by the way, I am a nurse" or "I am a doctor" or "I am a nurse practitioner", I typically acknowledge the statement right away. I say, "That's great. Where do you work, and in what capacity?" This generally gives the patient a few minutes to give a bit more information about the profession. In addition to hlping the patient become at ease, the process of disclosing the patient's professional medical background may also help the treating clinician obtain more information about what level of knowledge the patient may already have about the presenting ailment. This is very important because when the patient is a health care provider, the treating clinician must make every effort not to treat the patient as a complete novice but to expand on the patient's existing medical knowledge while correcting any misconceptions the patient may have. The treating clinician must strive to involve the patient's perspectives in arriving at the most appropriate medical plan of care.

Sometimes, I engage the patient in a general dialogue about the information that the patient disclosed about his or her profession. I avoid a lot of private chitchat and focus on information pertaining to the patient's profession. There are also times when the patient may not disclose specific details of work experience, and I simply mention generally known facts about the patient's stated profession. For example, a patient may mention that he works in a busy hospital with a particular population: mental health, pediatrics, oncology, or the elderly. My usually typical reaction is to find a response that highlights the rewards and challenges of working in such particular setting, or a response that highlights a common ailment in such settings.

This simple but empowering act takes only a few minutes to accomplish. It opens up room for a simple dialogue of interest between both parties, and it definitely goes a long way toward trust establishment between the treating clinician and the patient.

Many years ago, in my anticoagulation medical practice, I had a patient who was also a veterinarian and owned his vet practice. He was referred to me by his cardiologist for anticoagulation management. I will refer to this patient as "Dr. V." His initial consultation was on an early Tuesday morning. Upon arrival to my office, he appeared a bit uncomfortable as he sat down, and he said, "I'm glad to have finally made it to your office. I've needed help for quite some time in managing my Coumadin levels, and being a busy veterinarian does not help at all in watching what I eat." I looked at him and sensed an awkward tension developing. I knew I had to say or do something to break the ice and assist Dr. V to feel more at ease during the visit. Thankfully, I remembered that a neighbor of mine at that time had a dog with diabetes, and this dog required insulin administration for diabetes management. This concept of administering insulin injections to dogs had always been a fascination of mine, so I took this opportunity to casually mention it to Dr. V. The topic definitely piqued Dr. V's interest, and he informed me of the challenges of managing animal diabetes because animals lack the ability to verbalize symptoms that could signify low or high blood sugar levels. I nodded in agreement as I stated that animal owners actually run the risk of giving more than the required dose of insulin, especially when the animal is acutely ill with reduced appetite.

Dr. V responded that animals with very attentive owners tend to have less risk of glucose fluctuations, and the owner's attention and care for the animals is a great predictor of the animal's response to diabetic care. This dialogue with the patient took about five minutes, and as I proceeded to obtain a clinical history for the day's consultation, he appeared much more comfortable. He was very forthcoming with all the clinical information I needed to adequately manage his Coumadin dosing, lifestyle, and dietary patterns. By the end of the visit, I could sense the beginning of a meaningful clinician relationship with him.

I have found such visits to be some of my most enjoyable consultations, because these patients tend to give very thorough medical histories and can easily be engaged in a clinical conversation. It is important to note that the treating clinician should refrain from being overly analytical with the patient, who is also a health care provider. It's because many of these patients most likely have some idea of the various differential diagnosis associated with their presenting complaints, especially in the outpatient medical clinic settings. Rather, the treating clinician should endeavor to make the consultation process more of a partnership with the patient. Such patients usually come to the clinic with the expectation to listen and consider the treating clinician's view, while both patient and clinician explore other possible differential diagnosis in order to jointly arrive at the best options for treatment. Clinicians (especially new clinicians) should strive to avoid excessive nonclinical chitchat and keep the visit conversations to clinical points pertaining to the visit.

In conclusion, there is no magic strategy to establishing a trusting relationship with the patient who is also a medical provider, but a general guideline is that the treating clinician must find a means to create an invitation for a brief, friendly dialogue very early in the consultation. It is important not to ignore the initial statement that discloses the patient to be a medical provider. This is usually the most optimal time to begin a dialogue of interest. And sometimes, it may be the only chance a clinician gets to initiate an effective and productive clinician-patient relationship.

CHAPTER FIFTEEN

Communicating News of Terminal Illness to a Patient

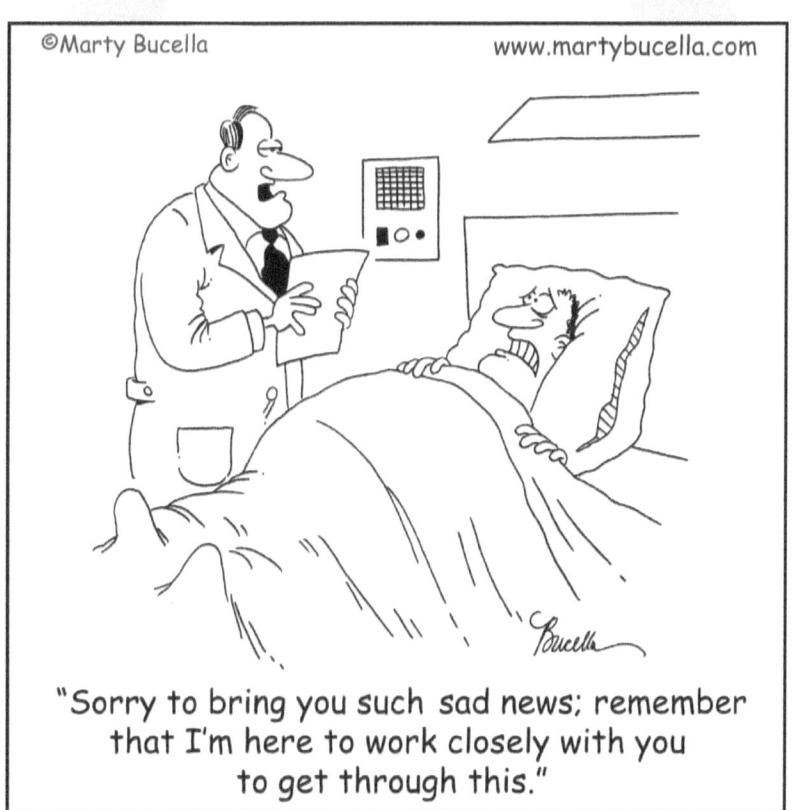
"Sorry to bring you such sad news; remember that I'm here to work closely with you to get through this."

Many patients who receive the unfortunate news of a terminal diagnosis may react differently. Communicating this report in an individualized basis is paramount to establishing a trusting relationship, because we all process information and express grief in different ways. It is natural for patients to systematically follow the five stages of the grieving process when informed of a chronic diagnosis or a debilitating illness such as cancer. These five stages are *denial*, *anger*, *bargaining*, *depression*, and *acceptance*. Some patients, however, may not typically display these five stages of the grieving process in the common sequence. They may flip in and out of each stage without following the stages in a linear fashion.[2]

It is important for the clinician to identify the patient's reactions and communicate appropriately during these stages of the grieving process, in order to establish a trusting and productive relationship with the grieving patient. In these early stages of the grieving process, the news may be very overwhelming, and the patient may go into a state of shock and denial as a means to initially cope with such devastating news. Patients may also shut down and refuse to communicate their fears and concerns to the clinician. The patient's lack of communication sometimes signifies shock and denial, and for some patients, it becomes a means of pacing overwhelming feelings of grief. Some patients may display immediate emotions of anger. It is important for the clinician to understand that beneath every emotion of anger that a patient displays, there is also an overwhelming feeling of pain. The patients may typically extend this anger to friends, loved ones, families, coworkers, and even to the clinician.

Occasional feelings of nonchalance may accompany this anger as the patient experiences an internal struggle to find answers to such commonly asked questions as, "Why me? What did I do to deserve this diagnosis?" The clinician should not be offended if the patient seems to zone in and out during conversations and struggles to

---

[2] David Kessler, "Because Love Never Dies: The 5 stages of Grief." Accessed April 16, 2016. http://grief.com/the-five-stages-of-grief.

accurately process and retain information. Clinician empathy is vital during these early stages while the diagnosis, plan of care, and treatment options are discussed with the patient. When possible, information may need to be reiterated during each visit because patients will need some time to process information as they come to terms with the diagnosis. In addition to having these discussions with the patient, the clinician should remember to focus on how the patient is faring with simple activities by asking questions that focus on various social and daily activities. For example, is the patient still in contact with friends and family? Is the patient currently working or did the patient stop working following the diagnosis? Is the patient still currently able to drive? Is the patient keeping up with his or her appearance? It is important to routinely review and discuss the patient's level of involvement with these basic daily life activities, and to encourage participation based on the patient's tolerance level. It certainly would be comforting for the patient to observe that in addition to monitoring disease progression and treatment options, the clinician also cares about the patient's daily life. This fosters trust development.

For some patients, disclosure of such devastating news like a terminal illness may cause them to experience overwhelming anxiety that increases over time. Such patients may become overly talkative and lack focus during consultation sessions with the clinician. Clinicians must be very sensitive to a patient's reactions and initiate a referral (if needed) for additional support to help the patient and family cope with a diagnosis of this nature. Note that it is only when a patient is finally able to experience less anxiety, and gradually begins to adequately process information and gain focus, that the patient will genuinely experience the five stages of the grieving process in sequence. In the following stage of the grieving process, *bargaining*, patients experience feelings of ambivalence as they struggle within themselves to obtain answers to questions as "If only I did this, this may not have happened", "What if I hadn't done this or that, this may not have happened, and things would have turned out differently," or "Oh, God, if you give me one more chance, I will do things differently."

Many patients may be open to discussions about the impact of spirituality as it pertains to their terminal illness. The clinician should be vigilant in identifying this need, and if comfortable with it, should be discussing it with the patient. Alternatively, the clinician can refer the patient to appropriate sources where this can be discussed (e.g., clergy, spiritual support groups). In all my years of interacting with my patients, as a born-again Christian, I have never shown any hesitancy in praying with my patients who request it. This stage typically gives way to the next stage of depression, where patients may experience a disconnection with daily life activities and are in a fog of intense sadness.

In the final stage of acceptance, patients become more aware of their current situation and finally come to terms with their new reality. Feelings of ambivalence are markedly diminished as many patients are ready to fight for their lives. Patients become more focused and retain more information as they fully explore treatment options and a plan of care with family, social support systems, and clinicians. This seems to be a stage where the sincerest communication with clinician takes place; patients are finally ready to bare it all and are at peace with the results of all treatment attempts. As a clinician, I would imagine that this is the point where clinicians should strive the hardest to become the most approachable for patients, because they're at their most vulnerable period in their lives.

Note that there is no specific time period assigned to each of these different stages of grieving. They are responses to the patient's feelings and can last from minutes to hours, days, or months. Clinicians should strive to maintain a positive outlook and give physical, emotional, and spiritual encouragement to all patients. This is important because it helps the patient to remain optimistic and maintain a trusting relationship with the clinician.

CHAPTER SIXTEEN

The Adolescent Patient

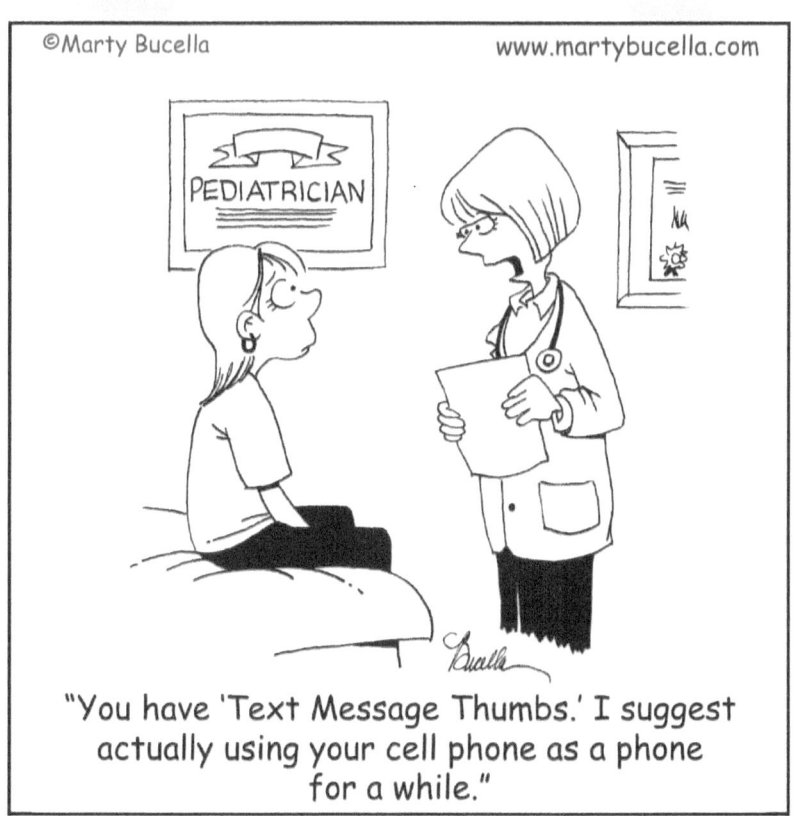

This is a very short chapter (probably one of the shorter chapters of this book) because with the appropriate tactics, it is not difficult to engage the adolescent patient in an open and honest clinical dialogue. With parental approval and permission from the adolescent patient, clinicians may be required to examine an adolescent patient in the absence of his or her parent. The adolescent patient is typically self-conscious and shy and may not readily divulge clinical information without adequate prompting on the clinician's part.

On the flip side, attempting to mask his or her true feelings or in order to deal with increasing anxiety, the adolescent patient may become overly talkative and display some lack of focus while narrating clinical history. The clinician must make every effort to put the adolescent patient at ease exceedingly early in the clinical visit. This is typically accomplished with a simple and pleasant questioning approach by the clinician to determine the adolescent's area of special interests. Any of these questions is an appropriate one to ask: "What grade are you in? Did you miss school today because of your illness? What's your favorite subject in school? What sports do you like to play?" Such questions create an atmosphere of general interest, and the adolescent patient (like any other patient) appreciates that the clinician is not only fixated on the presenting ailment but also has an interest in knowing a bit more about him or her.

This initial conversation with the clinician encourages the adolescent patient to concentrate on one particular topic at a time, which assists the patient to improve on overall focus and reduce anxiety. In addition, this approach encourages the patient to respond appropriately to the clinician's questions without much reservation during the history-taking process. In my practice, an adolescent patient may present to obtain a physical examination clearance to participate in sports activities. At the conclusion of such a visit, I always congratulate the patient for continuing with sports participation, which is great for overall health and well-being. I sometimes give a high-five greeting to those who proudly inform me of their accomplishments and the awards they've earned in their competitions. At the end of the visit, as I bid them farewell, I typically end with an upbeat remark like "Stay safe!"

This approach is very successful in developing a meaningful relationship with the adolescent patient, who then becomes eager to return to the clinician in the future for sports physical clearance and other acute medical visits.

Nonye Tochi Aghanya, MSc, RN, FNP-C

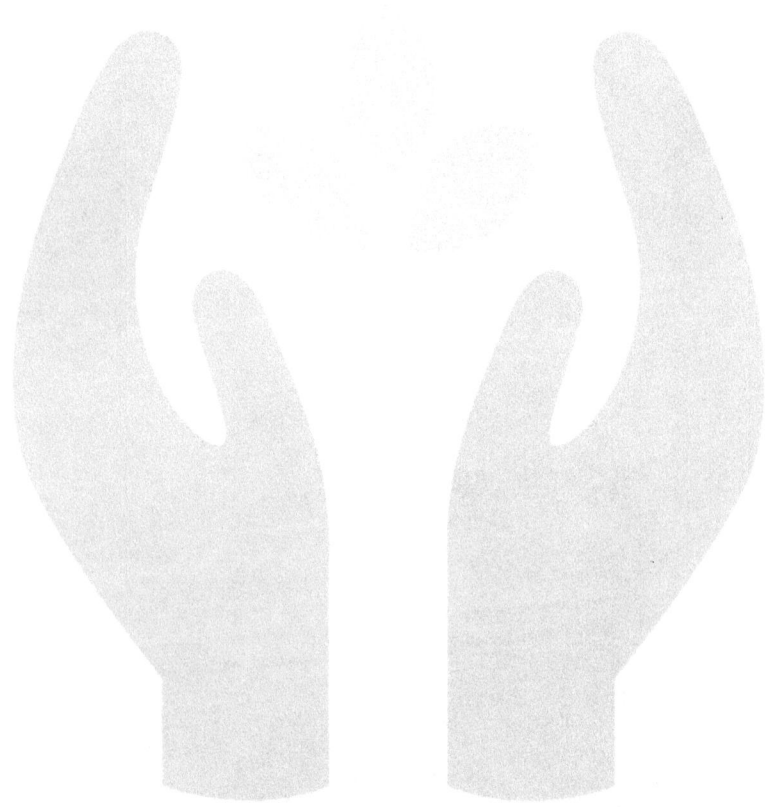

CHAPTER SEVENTEEN
The Medical Patient with a Mental-Health Challenge

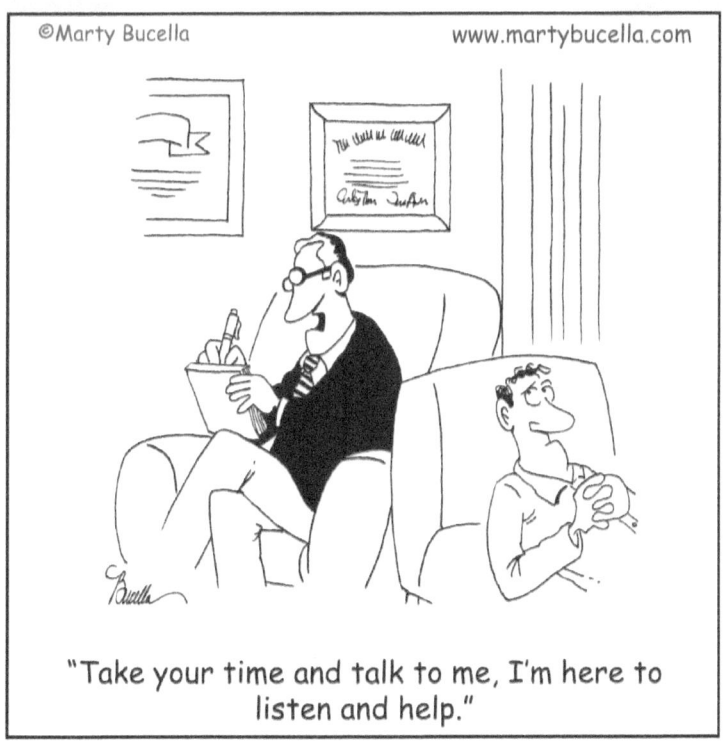

Clinicians may not have frequent encounters with this type of patient in an outpatient medical clinic setting. This is because patients with major psychological diagnoses typically have more routine consultation visits with those with specific specialties such as psychiatrists, psychologists, neuropsychiatrists, behavior therapists, and interventional therapists. These specialists tend to abide by their established and effective patterns of communication with the patients in their specific settings. However, some patients who present to the internal medical clinics for their general health management and episodic sick visits may have some established psychological medical diagnoses with some mental health-challenges that are managed by psychotropic medications and behavior therapy. Such patients may display underlying psychological behaviors during consultation visits with the clinician in the outpatient medical clinics.

Developing a trusting relationship with a patient who has a mental- health challenge can become quite an uphill battle if the clinician does not make an endeavor to gain the patient's trust during the initial visit. Many patients with psychological diagnosis already grapple with trust issues, and the clinician must implement a very strategic approach to develop trust in order to be successful in gaining the patient's trust. Through all my years of practice, I've found out that the most effective communication approach is redirection while showing empathy to the medical patient with a psychological diagnosis. What do I mean by that? With this group of patients, I typically do not implement my prior rule of "never underestimate the power of clinical knowledge." This digression from this rule is necessary because while communicating with a patient with a psychological diagnosis and mental-health challenge, clinicians should be cautious about disclosing a lot of information concerning the patient's medical health, disease process, plan of care, and medical tests during the initial consultation visit. There is more of a tendency for the patient to feel overwhelmed and tune out the conversation after a while, with the false perception that he or she is not being listened to and is only being told what to do.

A successful approach that I've implemented during initial visits with such a patient is to speak less and listen more. I typically encourage the patient to speak for most of the visit time (sometimes up to 80 percent) while I only speak to clarify any information that the patient narrates. I have noted that in many instances, the patient with a psychological diagnosis has a lot say. Some of the points and ideas that are verbalized are often clinically relevant history that will assist the clinician in building a clinical picture, which ultimately contributes to initiating the most appropriate medical plan of care. However, the general thought process and conceived ideas for such patients are in scattered bits and pieces, lacking the tendency to flow in cohesion.

One interesting observation that I've also made is that this patient usually has a perception that he or she could be halted by the clinician while attempting to give a narrative history. This perception creates an underlying anxiety that fuels the habit that many of these patients typically display: speaking very fast in an attempt to give full disclosure of past medical histories, patient interests, treatment plans, social and family histories, and fears and reservations—all in one very lengthy sentence! As noted before, this act is likely due to the patient's fear of being prematurely stopped by the clinician before the entire history is disclosed. Sometimes, there exists a belief by the patient that his or her opportunity to disclose an entire life history is primarily during the initial consultation, and such an opportunity may not present again in future visits. The combination of that thought process and an established psychological diagnosis makes for a patient who speaks so quickly that he or she stumbles on words, lacks focus, and exhibits flights of ideas and some memory lapses –making communication all the more frustrating for the patient and clinician.

I had a clinical consultation with a very well-educated patient who had an existing diagnosis of schizophrenia with manic tendencies. Because of his psychological diagnosis, he had visited quite frequently with his psychiatrists, and his resulting mood disorder, secondary to his diagnosis, was well controlled on psychotropic medications. He also frequently consulted other various medical specialists because of several underlying medical problems. He visited with an endocrinologist for his diabetes management, a pulmonologist for his diagnosis of chronic obstructive pulmonary disease, and some surgeons because of other minor surgical procedures he'd had a few years prior. He came to my practice with a common complaint of ear pain following a head cold. When I enquired about his medical history, he appeared very anxious and spoke so fast that he stumbled over his words. Seeing this, I gently asked him to take his time and tell me about his medical history because I needed to know the full history in order to make the best medical decision for him.

The look on this patient's face was priceless as he stated, "Wow, no doctor has ever said that to me before. Usually no one listens attentively to me because I have such a lengthy medical history from seeing so many different doctors." I assured him that I was listening and encouraged him to proceed, and with only occasional flights of ideas, he spoke for about 80 percent of the visit time, stopping intermittently to clarify any points per my request as I took down notes. Although he still spoke at a fast pace, he no longer stumbled over his sentences, and I observed that his anxiety was markedly reduced as he spoke. I obtained a very thorough history, performed a physical exam, and treated him for a minor bacterial infection. He was much more at ease and trusting during subsequent visits to the clinic.

In conclusion, although it is a daunting task at first, it is imperative that the clinician embrace this process with a great deal of patience with a patient who has a psychological diagnosis and mental-health challenges during his/her first few clinical visits. It is vital to create an atmosphere in which the patient feels at ease with the clinician. This is achieved when patients are given the opportunity to speak while the clinician listens attentively, and with the clinician interrupting only to clarify the patient's points. The clinician can gradually piece together a clinical picture. Don't be alarmed if this process seems to take up the entire visit time during the first few visits. It gets better with subsequent visits as a trusting relationship is gradually developed. Such patients are typically less anxious at subsequent visits and tend to disclose less medically irrelevant histories as their trust in the clinicians improves. This contributes to greater chances of effective medical management while curbing the patient's underlying psychological issues of trust, anxiety, self-doubt, and depression.

Nonye Tochi Aghanya, MSc, RN, FNP-C

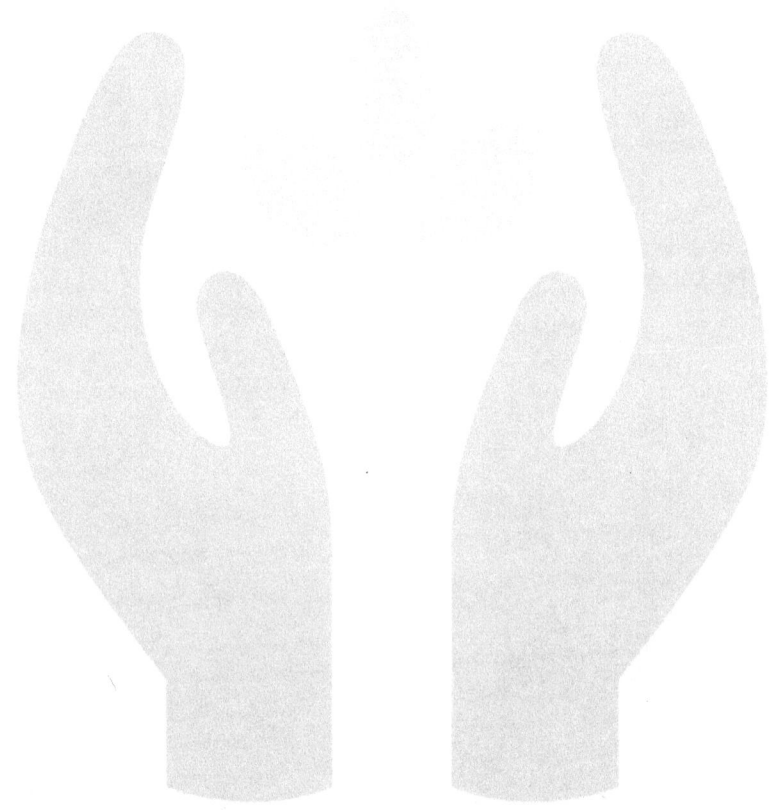

CHAPTER EIGHTEEN

Discussing Weight with the Obese Patient

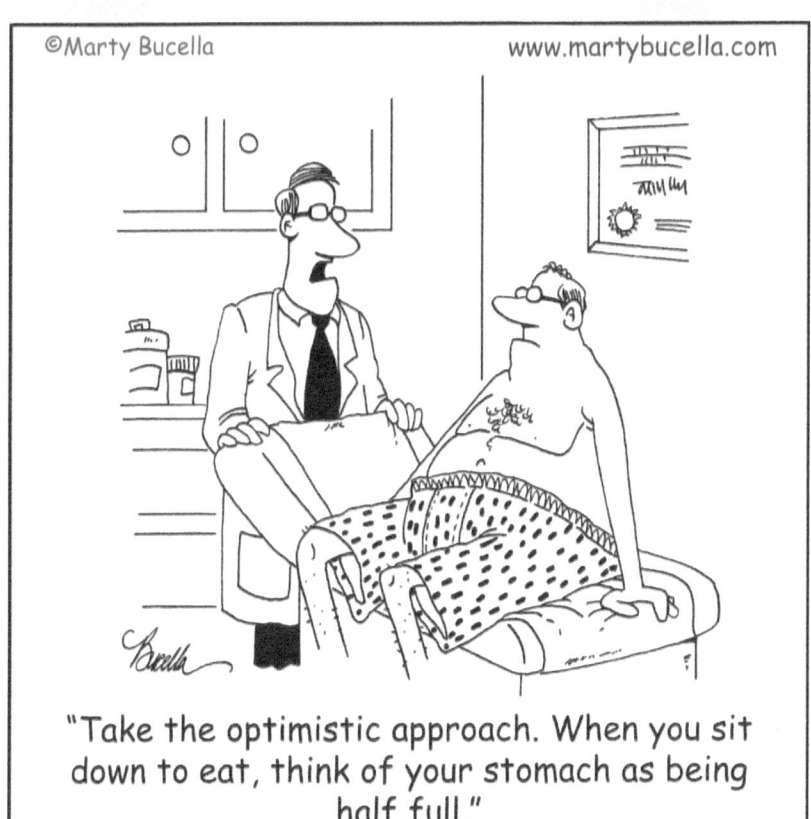

"Take the optimistic approach. When you sit down to eat, think of your stomach as being half full."

Communicating and building a trusting relationship with the obese patient, when conversation is centered on weight loss, is a unique process. It is important that the clinician understand that obesity is a stigmatized condition and has the potential to make the obese patient develop a defensive state of mind. Many patients may feel a sense of failure or even shame because of their past unsuccessful dietary and weight loss attempts.

An optimal approach to communicating with the obese patient is to encourage the patient to understand that the weight-loss process is a shared decision-making process between the clinician and the patient. This encourages the patient's full participation without withholding vital and detailed information that is necessary in developing a successful medical plan of care. During the initial visit with the clinician, providing the obese patient with weight loss dietary pamphlets and literature without further actions is not an effective move in developing a trusting relationship. Many obese patients have probably tried various diets in the past and have read numerous weight-loss plans and literature—which have likely proven unsuccessful. Giving the patient one more weight-loss pamphlet on the initial consultation visit is not a bright idea.

A better approach is to establish trust through honest communication while showing compassion to the patient first. The clinician may begin with a simple, open-ended question or comment. "I see from your notes that you have gained some weight in the past few years. What help can I offer you in your current attempts to lose weight?" Such a statement is an icebreaker for a topic that many patients find quite sensitive and would rather handle on their own terms. This statement also acknowledges that the patient may have tried unsuccessfully to lose weight but it still opens the line of communication, indicating that the clinician is available to explore other weight-loss options with the patient.

Many patients do not necessarily become obese from exclusively consuming large amounts of calories. But there often exists an underlying need for overconsumption of calories, and this behavior is the major identifiable risk factor for obesity. As clinicians, we know that it is very difficult to change a patient's behavior by repeatedly telling the patient what to do. Many clinicians do not also have the luxury of time for extensive, face-to-face meetings with patients to implement change within a short time period. However, all clinicians have the opportunity to acquire the necessary communication skills to create in an obese patient the desire to change those past habits and behaviors that have contributed to the patient's obesity. The million-dollar question is, "How can a clinician assist a patient to develop the desire for change?" A Medscape Article, "Obesity Management: Improving Outcomes," states that by engaging patients, several applicable frameworks for weight loss success were highlighted (Kushner et al. 2015).

There are the five as of frameworks to effective weight loss management (similar to five As of smoking cessation): ask, advise, assess, assist, and arrange. With this model, the clinician does not encourage behavior change by repeatedly telling patients to change their behaviors. Rather, the clinician attempts to promote patient engagement with a process that eventually leads to positive behavior changes with resulting weight loss (Alexander et al. 2011).

During this first phase of the process, it is important to Ask the patient and ascertain whether this is an important time to engage in a weight-loss conversation. If a patient is not mentally ready to take on the challenge of weight loss, the clinician's attempts will be futile as she proceeds to implement the rest of the process with little or no patient interest. If the patient gives an affirmative response and is ready to discuss weight-loss plans, the clinician must acknowledge this major step. Congratulating the patient on taking a positive step toward future health and well-being is a vital step in trust development. Such congratulatory action by the clinician is critical in ensuring that the second phase of the process, Advice, is perceived and accepted wholeheartedly by the patient. The clinician should bear in mind that many obese patients, in past quests for weight loss, have received plenty of advice that may not have helped them achieve success. In this phase of the process, the clinician's role is to tailor the specifics of health benefits as it directly relates to each obese patient. A typical statement by a clinician to an obese patient with hypertension could be, "Mr. J, it is great that you have decided to discuss your weight and available options for weight loss. Once we are able to identify areas in your life that we can make some changes to and once you begin to lose weight, I'm sure your blood pressure will greatly improve."

The third phase of the process, Assess, closely explores the patient's history. It involves honest clinician-patient conversations in an attempt to determine who the patient is. With honest interactions, this step reveals to the clinician what types of barriers and challenges the patient may have encountered with previous weight-loss attempts. In addition, the patient's food preferences, activity level, and social habits that may have contributed to weight gain are explored. This step of the process also creates the opportunity for the clinician to explore the patient's emotional perspective of what it means to lose and maintain a healthy weight. Some patients may view weight loss as an attempt to improve physical appearance and avoid the social stigma attached to being overweight. This is typical for patients who have struggled with being overweight for many years, including the preadolescent, adolescent, and young adult years. For these patients, it is important for the clinician to be empathetic during this phase of the process, so that the patient feels comfortable with sharing past painful experiences related to being overweight. This assists the clinician in obtaining the most pertinent information applicable to each patient prior to embarking on the fourth phase of the process.

During the *Assist* phase, the clinician has established that the patient is willing to lose weight. A useful tool that the clinician can implement in this phase is a motivational interview (Armstrong et al. 2011). Motivational interviewing is used to understand the patient's perspectives, build a partnership with the patient, and help the patient figure out how to overcome obstacles on his or her own. It focuses on the concept of ask, listen, and inform. It also emphasizes the importance of reflective listening. Motivational interviewing helps reduce patients' ambivalence because they are assured that the clinician is working very closely with them to implement and achieve their weight-loss goals. The clinician begins a partnership with the patient and discusses the pros and cons of maintaining current dietary and exercise habits. The clinician and the patient then tackle the pros and cons and prioritize what needs to be changed immediately and what would be most beneficial in preventing further damage to the patient's health. Motivational interviewing is a skill, and once a clinician acquires this skill and gets used to it, the clinician can understand the patient's readiness or ambivalence and what is most important to the patient regarding - a weight-loss initiative. It is important for the clinician to listen to the patient and then repeat or reflect back what the patient had said. This is reflective listening, and it's a great tool for the motivational interviewing process. Following a patient's statement, the clinician can reply, "I hear you say ……," "What do you think can you do to help you solve the problem?" Such an interactive statement enables the clinicians to isolate and elicit an action plan from the patient that can be improved on with input from both the patient and the clinician. Patients are more likely to comply with plans that are developed in an interactive manner.

With clinician's awareness of the patient's health and social habits, previous weight-loss attempts, and the current level of commitment for a healthy lifestyle, the final phase of the process is next. During the *Arrange* phase, the clinician helps the patient to develop a specific plan of action to achieve the weight-loss goal. This task should never be given to the patient to tackle alone; it continues to be a mutual effort between both patient and clinician. It may also involve patient's outreach to other external areas such as personal trainers or a gym membership. During this phase, the clinician can also incorporate the expertise of other disciplines such as dieticians, physical therapists, and nutritionists in order to better individualize the patient's weight-loss plan. This is the most appropriate phase to develop and review healthy lifestyle guides (literature, pamphlets, etc.) with patients, in order to provide them with the tools that would assist them in making smarter food choices and discuss the importance of embarking on regular physical exercise. In this phase, what you need to do is to have routine follow-ups to evaluate the patient's progress, reevaluate and modify the plan of care (if needed), and provide ongoing encouragement to the patient.

CHAPTER NINETEEN
The Electronically Savvy Patient

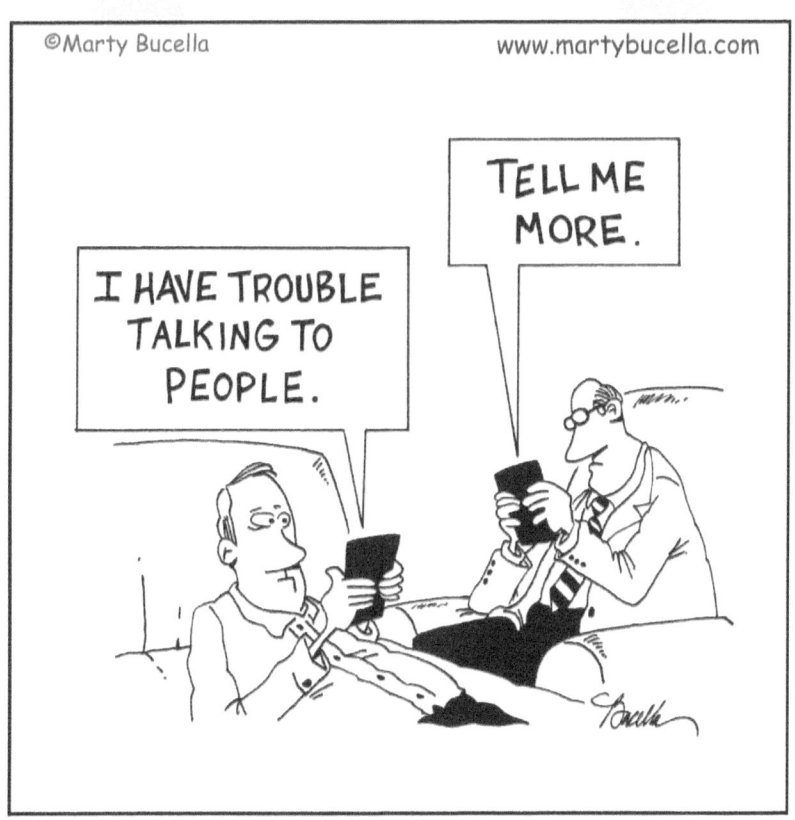

Do You Know You Can Do More with Your Electronic Devices?

The design of the electronic health record system (EHR) is gradually shifting from its initial predominant role of documenting and storing patient health information in easily accessible format and generating billing codes to a role of a more comprehensive design involving entering data and coordinating care for safer health care practice. More electronic health record developers are taking into account new sources of information, including data generated by mobile apps and genomic data. Although apps are not officially classified as medical devices, many patients who are more advanced with the use of technological devices have relied on different types of apps in monitoring and changing their behavior patterns. Personally, I could be considered a bit of an old-fashioned individual because I still have my flip phone from fifteen years ago. On some occasions, I would send and receive texts on my flip phone. There were no other features or applications on my flip phone, so I got an iPhone a few years ago to check my messages and download other useful apps for routine use.

However, I have observed that in recent times, more people use their electronic devices strictly as nonverbal communication tools (e.g., texting) and prefer to text families, friends, and colleagues rather than engage in face-to-face dialogue or verbal telephone conversations. Unfortunately, with excessive implementation of such nonverbal means of communication, an individual's personality could gradually erode as the individual relies heavily on such a mode of communication. With time, when this individual presents to a clinic as a patient, he or she is more likely to experience an increase in anxiety when engaging in face-to-face dialogue with a clinician. An important feature of innovative medical device is that it encourages shared decision-making between the patient and the clinician.

As a clinician, it is possible that with a simple clinic questionnaire, you can identify your patients who have access to innovative medical devices. The process of conducting surveys and having the patients complete simple questionnaires also informs and reminds patients of the versatile use for these devices, which assist in enhancing the medical care while promoting healthy and productive clinician-patient relationships. This is done while taking into account the best scientific evidence that is available and incorporating the patient's values and preferences (Pollak et al. 2010).

In order to broaden the practice scope and reach various populations, it is important that clinicians strive to become aware of the latest technology and obtain adequate response to common questions while maintaining a good understanding of the general functions of these medical technological devices. Given the clinicians' scope of practice, clinicians should not only be aware of what is available within that scope, but also what is generally applicable and not applicable to their patients. Even though studies show that it's not currently widely utilized, clinical data transfer via electronic apps is here to stay. It's vital that clinicians are receptive, keep an open mind, and talk to their patients about the types of data that would be useful in improving patient care. It is important to inquire about what apps patients are familiar with, and what apps they are more likely to use. Once identified, patients should be provided with data that will help them download the best apps to apply to their routine health management plans.

Some apps are primarily fitness and nutrition related, and they are used by patients on a daily basis. Data obtained from a *"Let's Walk"* activity app can provide information regarding patient's active or sedentary lifestyle, which can help in developing a targeted, personalized plan of care for the patient. There are various online sites that claim to have the most accurate data about patients' health and management plans. Findings from a P. Krebs and D. T. Duncan study regarding health app use among mobile phone owners in the United States suggest that a large number of the population do not use health apps, and that even those who use health apps are likely to stop using them. The authors noted that such findings suggest that app developers need to better address consumer concerns. Two major consumer concerns that were highlighted in the study were the cost of apps and the high burden of data entry (Krebs and Duncan 2015).

Accurately studying and understanding how to access and filter health information is a necessity for all clinicians who wish to implement an electronic health management system. This is also a vital step prior to discussing questionable online health information with the patients, as it helps the clinician provide direction on how patients can identify and apply reliable health care information from websites. This section provides some details on alternate studies that reveal the influence of other electronic features such as texting in the management of long-term, chronic diseases, as well as the influence of an electronic device app in modifying patients' behaviors and diet regimen. Getting patients to properly manage their long-term, chronic diseases remains a challenge because of poor adherence in long-term therapies, which is primarily a result of complexities with some of the current traditional interventions to improve adherence (Thakkar et al. 2016).

In the *Journal of American Medical Association,* an article headed by Jay Thakker reports that the results of a meta-analysis of randomized clinical trials show that texting can improve drug adherence for chronic diseases. Texting may be a more scalable solution than other interventions, such as apps that require a certain kind of device and software. A patient with a diagnosis of congestive heart failure may receive a weekly text reminder to monitor weight and report the value to the clinician. A patient with atrial fibrillation who takes Coumadin and is on a self-monitoring regimen for checking the international normalized ratio values may receive a weekly, biweekly, or monthly text reminders to check the INR level and report that level to the clinician for Coumadin dose adjustments. Unlike other diverse apps, texting technology is well established and can be used on almost any mobile phone. However, it is noteworthy to indicate that at the conclusion of the study in the JAMA article, the authors pointed out that text messaging is a low-cost technology that has the potential to become widespread. More extensive testing and development is needed to determine whether it has enduring and long-lasting benefits for the patient—and whether it is worth investing in.

Other clinical studies that were conducted show that patients who were involved in these studies were able to modify their behaviors and diet regimens with the use of appropriately applied health apps. As mobile technology becomes increasingly available to more people than ever before, it affords a scalable platform to extend continuing support for healthy behavior change pervasively into the environment with the potential to improve the health of the population (Spring et al. 2012). This study by Spring actually demonstrated that a smart phone app can be useful in implementing sustainable behavior changes. According to the study results, the basic principle is that patients need something that gives them a visible goal, causes them to self-monitor, and gives them feedback (e.g., activity tracker apps, food tracker apps). Participants in this study recorded their food intake and wore an accelerator that measured their activity levels. Data obtained were transmitted to a behavior coach. Participants received monetary compensation if they met certain goals. Interestingly, the study report showed that even after the participants were no longer paid to perform these behaviors, they maintained about half of the behavior improvement.

Through the practice of an ever-expanding concept of precision medicine, the clinician can discover how to review and apply the patient's collected data for more optimal medical management. It affords the clinician the opportunity to begin to learn more about the patient's lifestyles and incorporate this into a targeted clinical decision-making process. This is because most of our health status is determined by our lifestyles, not our genes or the environment. The clinician can potentially learn specifics about how a patient's lifestyle translates to the existence or nonexistence of a medical condition and patient longevity (Fiore et al. 2015). This is truly a remarkable correlation that is worth exploring, and it is another mode of interaction to further enhance an existing clinician-patient relationship.

Nonye Tochi Aghanya, MSc, RN, FNP-C

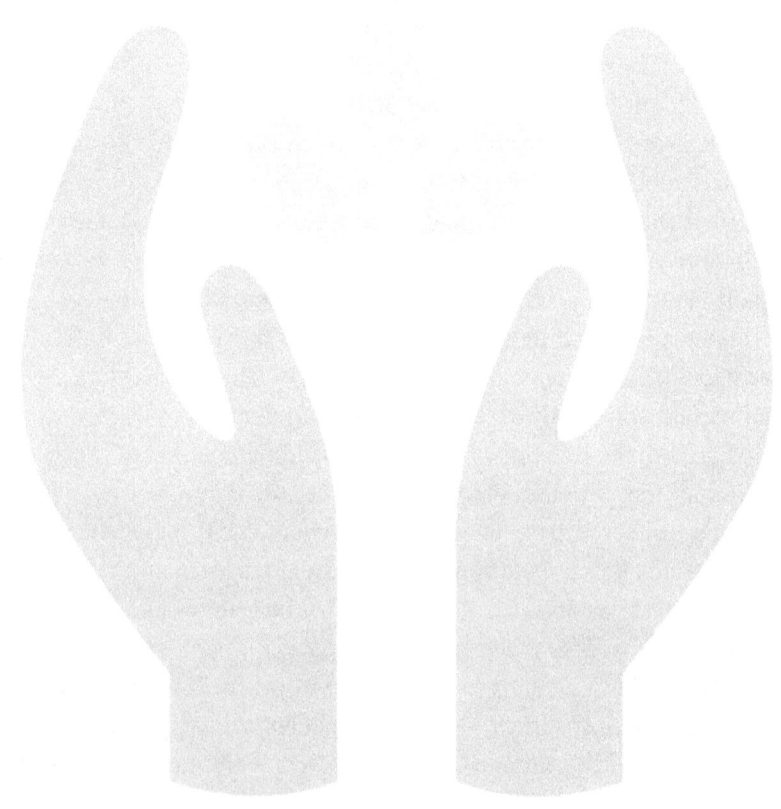

CHAPTER TWENTY

The Defiant Patient (the Aging Parent)

This chapter is very personal to me, and I'm sure that there are many families out there that face the challenge of dealing with aging parents. Please allow me to say this: my dad is a defiant patient. In his mid-eighties, my dad was very strong willed, caring, and positively minded and he remains the most opinionated individual that I've ever met. He has a sharp sense of right and wrong and is very much cognitively intact. He has always maintained a higher level of independence than the average elderly person, and he knows not to push boundaries that would become detrimental to his health and well-being. As an ex-military man, he has always maintained an athletic built with a strong sense of focus by engaging in consistent exercise activities and healthy dietary habits.

As a retired colonel and senior army officer, Dad always displayed a "can do it all" attitude. Looking back at my childhood and adult years, I can say that I can't recall any obstacles that he did not seem to overcome. At age seventy-five, Dad could still do ten to twenty push-ups each day, take leisure walks, and drive his 2010 Corolla around the neighborhoods to stores, the church, and community events. He was quite independent and was still very much in control of his day-to-day activities.

Although he retired many years ago from the Nigerian army,

conversations with Dad always reminded me of his status as a top commander in the military barracks. He was quick to give orders and maintained control of most conversation topics. He commanded attention and respect and was very respectful of everyone he came across. He diligently kept his doctor's appointments and religiously followed all the doctor's orders. He kept up with daily news information through daily Internet searches, and he always asked about his grandchildren. At age seventy-seven, Dad was diagnosed with glaucoma. In addition to other medications he was taking, he needed to instill eyedrops as part of his medical management routine. Dad was very meticulous with his eye drops administration and never missed his scheduled routine. With his eye sight still intact, he maintained his simple, independent lifestyle.

On a sunny afternoon in the summer of 2012, just after Dad's eighty- first birthday, I visited him at home. As I sat in his living room reading a book, he came and stood by the door. "Have you seen my glasses?" he asked.

I looked around the room and saw them on the table in the center of the room. "They're right there on the table," I said.

"Where?" he asked as he looked at the table. "Right there," I said while pointing at the table.

"I don't really see it," he said as he walked to the table. When he got closer to the table, he exclaimed, "Oh, there it is!" With some prior similar episodes that alluded to Dad's deteriorating eyesight, the family became quite concerned following this recent episode. We realized that Dad's sight may be worse than we'd thought.

As a family unit, we had numerous conversations with Dad and verbalized our concerns regarding the need for him to stop driving. He was quite upset at the family's suggestions and remarked that his independence was being taken from him. He said that he was very capable of driving, provided he continued to follow his doctor's orders and instill his glaucoma eyedrops. He wanted to maintain control of his choices regarding his daily living activities and was not psychologically ready to give up control. For individual and public safety concern, the family made a unified decision to withhold his car keys, and we made other transportation arrangements for Dad and Mom to fulfill their daily activities. More conversations with Dad did not help him accept the reason for this decision—they only fueled his anger. I observed that Dad's demeanor gradually changed from that of a warm, caring man to bitterness and frustration.

As the clinician in the family, other family members turned to me to "speak some sense into Daddy." There was definitely a mounting tension in the family as Dad became increasingly bitter about the family decision. I remember repeatedly having the same conversation with him without obtaining the effect I wished to achieve. I wanted Dad to agree with the family decision to take the keys from him and not be left with a feeling that his control and dignity were taken away from him. "You are still very strong, Daddy, and we love you very much. We want you to be around for many more years, but your eyesight is getting worse. It's no longer safe for you to drive anymore," I would say. Daddy would smile sadly and walk away. I knew that even though he understood the logic of our intentions, he was not ready to accept the fact that he was giving up control. I thought to myself, *I have to do something else. There must be a way to reach Daddy and make him understand that the family is not deliberately trying to take away his privileges. We have his best interest at heart to keep him and the public safe.*

The defiant patient is sometimes quite conscious about his health and is diligent with implementing healthy lifestyles to promote health and well-being. However, just like my dad, there could exist an independent mind-set that leads to a false sense of control, which later becomes detrimental to the individual's future well-being. As a clinician, I knew that I owed it to the public, my family, and my dad to explore the reasons why he was adamant in giving up his driving independence. I had to find a better way of communicating with Dad to get him to voluntarily surrender his car keys and ultimately come to terms with the loss of his driving independence.

In 2004, Dad wrote a book titled *Behind the Screen*. In this book, he gave a detailed account of his time in the Nigeria army as a colonel. As a busy mother, I had always found the 170-page book of war events a bit of a cumbersome task to read in its entirety. I usually skimmed over the pages. But when faced with this family dilemma, I knew I had to explore the contents of this book in order to determine the events that may have contributed to making my dad the defiant patient that he had become in his much later years.

As an army major and senior army officer in the Nigeria-Biafra war from 1967 to 1970, Dad commanded many groups of junior officers and soldiers who carried out his orders. He was always in control of events. He overcame many obstacles during those years via his sharp wit, focus, and dedication to a life of strict discipline and independent way of thinking. He had to come up with ideas and solutions to problems in order to command respect and remain in charge. This was a necessary step to keeping his troop of soldiers safe during the dangerous events of war. Following his retirement, as an electrical engineer he went on to build a traffic light system, and he had many employees who worked for him.

When I concluded with reading his book, I said to myself, "Wow, now I get it. I know how to speak to Daddy and achieve a breakthrough." I realized that Dad "just didn't get it," or stating that Dad was just being stubborn, selfish, or inconsiderate was not a productive approach. It could only deepen the bitterness within the family unit. Dad was not being stubborn; he simply did not know how to make the connection that even though his mind was still sharp and he was cognitively intact, his eyes were failing him. He was stuck in the mind-set of being a warrior who could overcome this challenge, as he often had in the past.

Early one morning, after I read Dad's book, I sat down with him and told him that I had finally read his book in its entirety. He was pleased to hear that, and I told him that I finally understood why it was difficult for him to give up control of driving independently. I reminded Dad that at his current age of eighty-four years old, and even with naturally declining health, he was still a warrior to the family. He did not need to continue to prove to himself, or to anyone else, that he was in complete control at all times. It was okay for him to seek assistance, and we were eager to offer assistance because we loved him and did not want him to risk hurting himself or anyone else by continuing to drive. Finally, I looked at him and said with tear-filled eyes, "Daddy, it's okay. You have to give up control. It's the right thing to do."

Dad looked at me and then lowered his head for a moment, as though he was lost in deep thought. After a few minutes, he looked up with a resolved facial expression, and as he made eye contact with me, he slowly nodded his head in agreement. I knew at that moment that my dad finally got the message. The look of defiance, anger, fear, animosity, and betrayal was gone from his eyes. He had come to terms with the natural aging process, which involves the gradual decline of health. He had made peace with the fact that withholding his car keys was not done to humiliate, punish, or diminish his role as a father; it was an act of love for him.

As a daughter of an aging parent, I felt compelled to write this chapter because I have also witnessed many patients with similar personalities in my years of practice. Sometimes, families of aging parents deal with so much opposition from the defiant patients as the patients are faced with the struggles of giving up their independence. My dad gave me his word that he had accepted the decision to give up his car keys with no remorse, but as a clinician, I knew that Dad had always maintained control of most aspects of his life, and he may still struggle with moments of regret for giving up driving. I knew he needed reinforcement from someone else who was in a position of authority to him. In addition to having this heart-to-heart conversation with Dad, I reached out to his clinician and requested that his primary doctor have a conversation with him to reinforce the need to implement this driving restriction. I realized that Dad would heed the advice of his doctor, because just as he was quick to give orders, he was also quick to take orders from those he considered to be in positions of authority.

There are different protocols in medical clinics regarding the most appropriate time to prevent the aging patient from driving. Some of these protocols may involve the patient's care provider notifying the Department of Motor Vehicles for driving restrictions because of the patient's deteriorating health. Families should also seek the advice of their elderly parent's clinician in determining the most appropriate course of action when it is deemed unsafe for an aging parent to independently operate a vehicle.

As always, it is important for the clinician to take some time and explore the defiant patient's background with both the patient and family. Any information regarding the patient's role in the family unit, as well as past employment (such as retired educators, chief executives, and retired military veterans for example) are invaluable information needed by the clinician to initiate the most appropriate conversational topics with the patient. This will assist the patient to come to terms with his or her fears and reservations about giving up control and independence.

The underlying roots of a patient's behaviors (especially the elderly) can be determined during this exploratory process, and the most appropriate communication approach typically emerges afterward. I have found out that in past encounters with such patients, the most effective communication approach was always directly related to the patient's life experiences. Every effort made to get the patient's perspective on his or her life experiences would help improve communication. It is unproductive to view the defiant patient as a "stubborn old man; selfish and stuck in his way." These characterizations limit the chance of exploring and attaining the underlying reasons for the defiant patient's behavior, and they do not help promote a productive clinician-patient relationship.

I DEDICATE THIS CHAPTER
TO MY DAD, MY HERO.

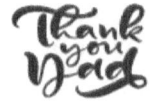

Rest in God's Perfect Peace, dad (1932-2020) ♥

CHAPTER TWENTY-ONE

The "Normal" Patient

Who is the normal patient? In my opinion, the normal patient is nonexistent. The term *normal* is a relative term and denotes certain characteristics that may be viewed as normal by one individual—but may very well seem abnormal to another individual. The question of normalcy creates strange paradoxes during clinical consultation. Origins of emotions such as love, fear, trust, and empathy play significant roles in determining the behavior and traits of our patients. Each of us possesses various traits and diverse characteristics that make us unique as individuals. The beauty of creation is found in the diversity of these traits. Knowledge of each individual's unique traits and characteristics is essential to forging meaningful clinician-patient relationships and ultimately improving communication in health care.

When a clinician fails to invest some time in really getting to know a patient, this creates the risk of a gradual stripping of the patient's unique traits and characteristics which could inadvertently force the patient to conform to a certain societal behavioral standard to make the clinician feel comfortable. In response, patients can sometimes become easily anxious, stoic, irritable, and easily forgetful in the presence of the clinician. They can also display a nonchalant attitude resulting in noncompliance with treatment plans. As clinicians, we should strive not to deny our patients the opportunity of assisting them to become their true selves, or else we will miss the chance of having an honest and productive clinician-patient interaction. It is our responsibility as clinicians to identify our patient's traits and unique characteristics in order to appropriately tailor our style of interaction to all diverse personalities that we encounter daily. Our patients will thank us and really mean it!

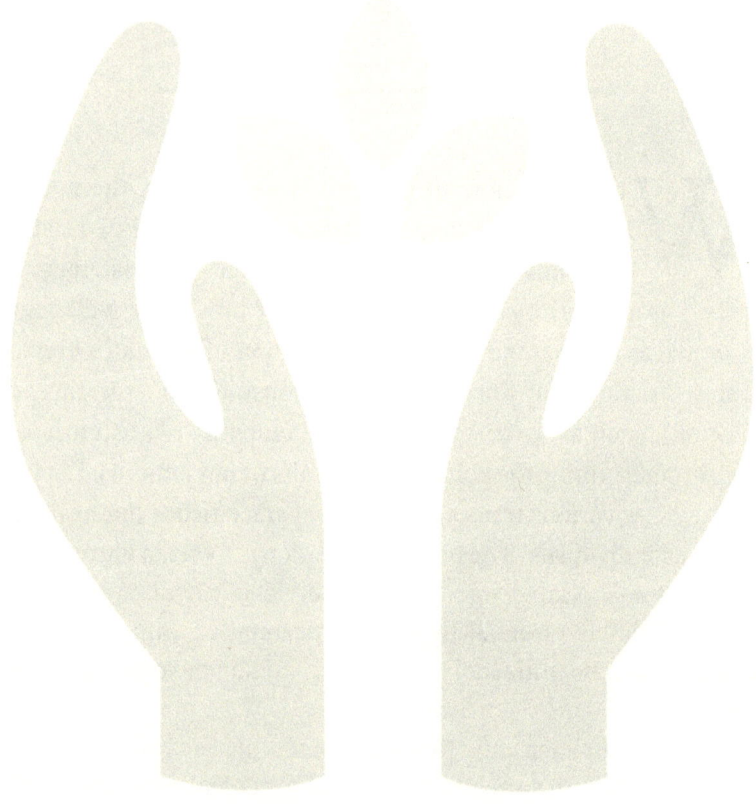

CHAPTER TWENTY-TWO

Review of Empirical Studies

Author, Nonye Tochi Aghanya's below report originally appeared in the *Transdisciplinary Agora for Future Discussions Journal* ISSN 2643-4938 (ONLINE) Volume Two Issue Two: August 2020

Evolution of Fear in Healthcare Management: Analyzing Influences of Communication Skills for Trust Development

Abstract

Quality healthcare requires practitioners who possess the technical competence and communication skills for not only gathering and transferring information to patients but also for developing trust with patients in the process of clinical consultation. The study used discourse analysis to identify how poor communication skills significantly contribute to the mistrust experienced between patients and healthcare providers/clinicians. The study identified various professional practice gaps in existence such as clinicians/healthcare providers who are unaware of different scenarios that warrant the application of specific styles of soft skills of communication while interacting with patients who present with different attitudes, characteristics or personal attributes. Education is needed to provide a better understanding of the several factors that contribute to these presenting attitudes, capable of building a wedge and creating mistrust between patients and healthcare providers/clinicians.

Keywords:
Opinionated Patient, Dependent Patient, Communication Skills, Suspicious Patient, "Normal" Patient

Introduction

In 2013, the author underwent a major abdominal surgical procedure which was debilitating. She was out of work for five months (See Photo 1). With immense gratitude to God, she has recovered and in excellent health today. However, during these five months of recovery in 2013, the surgery experience created many dependencies on family members and healthcare providers. In addition to visits to the primary care doctor, there were also visits to other specialists such as cardiologist, gynecologist, urologist and general surgeons to complete what seemed to be a series of never-ending medical examinations, tests, scans, and other diagnostic studies.

These underlying emotions and anxieties can eventually manifest as several kinds of patient behaviors and attitudes during a clinical visit. Aghanya (2016) agrees that clinicians could perceive various behaviors as overly curious, rude, dismissive, absurd, or downright bizarre. She posits that effective communication, especially in the healthcare sector, is essential for the well-being of patients and helps in the process of recuperation. Communication is the process of sharing meanings, ideas and services which must be interactive for effectiveness. Effective communication is, however, proactive when the communicator possesses adequate communication skills.

Tips for Effective Communication: A Vital Tool for Trust Development

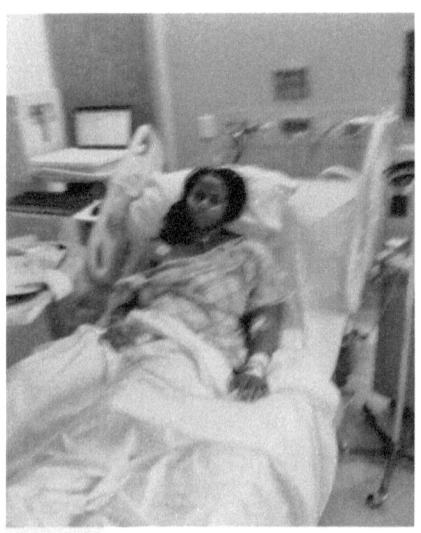

Photo 1: A patient in hospital

The need for a study which addresses this vital component of healthcare practice was realized following this personal experience of the author as a patient in the healthcare system. It was further substantiated after the review of various articles and research studies which explore the effects of empathy or compassionate interactions on patient care and its correlation if any, to the rate of clinician burnout. Many articles, journals, books, and presentations highlight various aspects of communication in healthcare but fail to identify or explore the factors that contribute to the formation or hindrance of a productive and trusting relationship between the patient and clinician. There are no studies identified which address the methodological management of fears/anxieties with strategic communication styles for various patients' attitudes/emotions.

Various studies highlight the evidence that whenever healthcare providers/clinicians are compassionate and strive to make more genuine connections with patients, they are happier and feel more fulfilled in their roles as this helps to reduce the risks of provider burnout. However, given that compassion is best implemented as an act, it became imperative to explore the etiology and effects of anxieties in healthcare and more importantly how healthcare providers/clinicians can strategically apply the soft skills of communication to improve the chances of delivering compassionate care to establish trust with patients.

The Problem
The author, who is also a clinician is familiar with the uncertainties of a clinical recovery process and the existence of such knowledge typically invoked substantial levels of fears and anxieties. Constantly grappling with several levels of anxiety and physical pain, this experience ultimately started to affect daily mood and outlook in life. It was a humbling experience which revealed that many, if not all patients in the healthcare system, experience different levels of anxiety/fear due to the feeling of not knowing what would be the outcome of any clinical situation they were in. "The unknown" can create feelings of crippling fear for some patients and others; can create moments of doubt, confusion, awkwardness (sometimes shown by misplaced smiles and laughter), irritation, and even bitterness. Ascertaining the relevance of communication skills in overcoming this kind of fear is, therefore, the main thrust of this research.

Method & Significance of Study
The study deployed discourse analysis to investigate the role and effectiveness of communication in healthcare. Findings and knowledge emanating from this study will help to provide strategies to healthcare providers/clinicians for active engagement apt which can help them build trust with patients especially those who present to healthcare settings with fears and anxieties due to underlying emotions such as anger, suspicions, dependence, defiance, feeling overwhelmed, talkative, sad, proud, opinionated, skeptical and so on. Irrespective of patients' attitude and countenance, utilizing strategic communication skills to transfer information from the healthcare provider should be done in a way that helps to allay patients' underlying fears and promote patients' understanding. Most importantly, it should encourage the adherence to the recommendations of the healthcare provider/clinician.

This educational information applies to various levels of healthcare practices such as primary prevention plans, education regarding disease and ailment management, prevention of hypertension, diabetes, obesity, smoking cessation plans; secondary prevention plans which include effectively communicating to patients the measures that lead to early diagnosis and prompt treatment of their diseases. And finally, tertiary prevention plans which include the most appropriate ways to empathetically engage with patients as healthcare providers/clinicians attempt to improve the quality of life of patients with terminal illnesses should be adopted. It is achieved by appropriately relaying information regarding treatment and prognosis of existing ailments and discussing the best ways to reduce symptoms of existing chronic diseases.

The helpful resources gained from this study originate from critical analysis of peer reviewed research articles and various studies, including thirty years of author's clinical experiences in diverse healthcare settings. The findings of this study would make a great teaching/learning tool in educational institutions such as medical/dental/nursing schools and healthcare practice settings such as medical clinics, emergency health clinics, hospitals, retail clinic, and urgent care clinics.

Literature Review

In recent times, an attempt to make sense of the correlation between the impact of fear on behaviors and life outlook, the works of various philosophers and their interpretations of fear were explored. Reading Dr Michael Fishers (2015) publication, "Educating Ourselves: A Lovist or Fearist Perspective", it was fascinating to note that his introductory paragraph detailed his observation as a Fearist, about the correlation between how we live our lives and how we educate ourselves. Fisher (2015) went on further to ask this vital questions: What exactly is fear? How does it evolve, and who gets to define it accurately? Can any single definition be all inclusively contained especially given the evolving human nature/views/opinions? Sometimes, there are even evolving philosophical views.

The healthcare atmosphere is an emotionally charged one,

capable of inducing various levels of anxieties/fears. We live in an emerging world of technological advancements where healthcare providers/clinicians are required to assess patients' histories adequately, arrive at a diagnosis, and provide treatment plans in a fast-paced environment. Such expectation is especially true in rapid care delivery settings such as walk-in medical clinics, retail clinics, and emergency room clinics. It seems to be a more difficult task for the healthcare provider/clinician to rapidly establish a rapport with the anxious/fearful patient while simultaneously assessing and developing a treatment plan with the patient.

Healthcare providers/clinicians need to realize that patients often heavily interpret the quality of their medical care based on the emotions that they most often experienced during their clinical interactions with healthcare providers. To successfully build trust with patients, healthcare providers/clinicians must therefore, develop a unique approach in communicating with every patient. The clinician-patient relationship can be a simple or complex one depending on the clinician's approach to allaying patient's anxieties/fears and establishing an enduring relationship. It is unwise to assume that a productive relationship is achievable without much input from both parties. Just as in every other relationship, there needs to be more effort made by the healthcare provider to relationship building because he/she is the figure of authority who guides the flow of the consultation.

A wrong move is when healthcare providers rely entirely on patients to set the tone of a consultation visit and control the visit flow pattern. Due to the patient's underlying fears, many patients expectantly look to healthcare providers to set the tone of the visit. Most patients would respond quickly and positively to a friendly tone from the healthcare provider/clinician. Many patients would also prefer to quickly establish this rapport than fidget in fear/anxiety in the clinician's presence for the duration of the visit. Healthcare providers/clinician must take advantage of this common patient expectation and apply it strategically to help allay the patient's fears and gain their trust. There is no disputing the fact that when people feel at ease and less fearful, they retain more information disclosed to them. This process of trust development between both parties requires a delicate balancing act. The division of race, ethnicity, and culture may be reflected in the health of the people in a community, society or nation. For instance, in the United States, despite recent progress in overall national healthcare delivery, disparities continue in the rising incidence of illness and death among African Americans, Latino/Hispanics, Native Americans, Asian Americans, Alaska Natives, and Pacific Islanders as compared with the United States population as a whole.

Various patient perspectives and mistrust of standard healthcare practices may emanate from the knowledge of such historical events as the 1932 Tuskegee study of black men which was unfairly conducted without adequate study disclosure or informed consents from study participants. There could be a result of increasing fears, anxieties, and mistrusts from the population/race most affected by the memories of such unfortunate study events (https://www.cdc.gov/tuskegee/timeline.htm). Healthcare practices (including communication process) must, therefore, be reflective of cultural sensitivities, perceived underlying fears and reservations emanating from historical events in various communities. Although subtle at times, culture does play a significant impact on the provision of appropriate healthcare services. Acknowledging, recognizing, and addressing these complexities will help facilitate learning and trust promotion between the healthcare providers/clinicians and patients. It is highly attainable irrespective of background, culture, ideologies, attitudes, and individualities.

Another philosopher with a breathtaking view is Osinakachi Akuma Kalu (Kalu, 2018). He argues that the necessary foundation of philosophy is rooted in problem-solving. His suggestion is congruent with the theory of evolution of fear in healthcare. Kalu (2018) assumes that identifying the roots of common fears of patients and healthcare providers/clinicians is the key to developing strategies for minimizing fears and anxieties that commonly exist in various societies. She posits that going further to develop resources that teach the necessary communication skills will help to avert these common fears experienced in healthcare settings. Kalu (2018,

53-54) further touched on the role of fear in the human struggle by identifying fear as a great motivator which is not typically self-contained but instead manifests as an external factor which when perceived, motivates one to react. How we choose to direct these emotions that conjure up within us due to external fears is a significant determinant of whether our fears/anxieties shall either control or not control our lives.

Another exciting opportunity was the review of another philosopher's work, Professor Desh Subba, who has detailed some interesting observations of fear from a positive perspective (Subba, 2014). He believes fear gives an interpretation of both life and the world. According to (Subba, 2014), *Fearism* exists as a theory and in order to study *Fearism*, there is a need to study all aspects of fear, its causes, and effects, how it has embedded into the societal values and affecting our behaviors and attitudes (our essence, our being). Subba (2014, p. 52) also indicates that fear comes from the human mind and while the existence of fear precedes essence, a combination of exterior and interior factors generates fears. Applicable to the theory of *Fearism* in healthcare, patient's awareness of clinical diagnosis and prognosis can either create feelings of uncertainties, despair, fears or anxieties and can create an innate commitment for the patient to battle the disease bravely. The author argues that knowing a patient's mindset helps the healthcare provider/clinician to engage strategically, which contributes to some tranquility amidst an otherwise chaotic moment.

In essence, the moment a healthcare provider/clinician is faced with an unfortunate health experience, common fears/anxieties is felt by patients. It is usually a life-changing experience that spurred into action and the development of resources for improving communication patterns that help alleviate patients' and healthcare providers' fears/anxieties in various healthcare settings.

Review of Empirical Studies
The following studies were reviewed to give an empirical undertone to this study:

Empathy decline and its reasons: a systematic review of studies with medical students and residents: In this study, the results of reviewed studies, especially those with longitudinal data, suggest that empathy decline during medical school and residency compromises striving toward professionalism and may threaten health care quality. Theory-based investigations of the factors that contribute to empathy decline among trainees and improvement of the validity of self-assessment methods are necessary for further research. (https://www.ncbi.nlm.nih.gov/pubmed/21670661).

Teaching empathy to medical students: an updated, systematic review: The findings of this study suggest that educational interventions can be useful in maintaining and enhancing empathy in undergraduate medical students. Also, it highlights the need for multicenter, randomized controlled trials reporting long-term data to evaluate the longevity of intervention effects. Defining empathy remains problematic though which is why the authors called for conceptual clarity to aid future research (https://www.ncbi.nlm.nih.gov/pubmed/23807099).

To add to conceptual clarity, Aghanya (2021) in her book, *"Tips for Effective Communication: A vital tool for Trust Development in Healthcare "* provides several practical tips that healthcare providers/clinicians can implement during consultation visits with patients that will help to alleviate patient's fears and anxieties. It explores the etiology of how various underlying fears and anxieties can manifest as patient's attitudes and behaviors which might become deterrents to the establishment of trust and relationships between patients and healthcare providers.

The importance of identifying these unique characteristics and implementing strategic communication styles can never be overemphasized. Healthcare providers/clinicians need to refrain from using a one-size-fits-all communication approach for all patient encounters because people have different personalities, backgrounds, and characteristic. They perceive and react differently to the same information presented to them. To attain long lasting trust development through active interaction, the healthcare provider/clinician must implement a communication style specifically tailored to each patient's personality, attitude, individuality, and background. Having known a patient's mindset, being, or essence can help a clinician to engage strategically aiding tranquility amidst an otherwise chaotic moment of life.

Findings, Conclusion & Recommendation

The review of literature has shown that communication is vital in overcoming and managing fear among patients of every category. The finding buttressed the relevance of possessing communication skills by health care workers. The study concludes that communication skills are needed for effective communication in healthcare. It helps overcome fear among patients. The study recommends the adoption of the contents of Aghanya's (2021) *"Tips for Effective Communication: A vital tool for Trust Development in Healthcare."* It gives the communication tips for allaying fears/anxieties for various scenarios regarding patients' attitudes/behaviors.

Aghanya (2021) argues that when one interacts with patients and encounters various attitudes, there are more appropriate times to implement either one or more of the communication styles listed in the below paragraphs. While utilizing this book as a resource in the medical/nursing educational curriculum, students would become empowered in learning the skills to assist patients to feel comfortable in their presence. She believes that students will learn when to effectively implement communication styles such as maintaining more constant eye contact versus temporarily avoiding eye contact (to give patients the chance to establish a train of thought pattern), and when to speak softly versus loudly (to create a tranquil environment).

It will also help them understand when to use open versus close-ended questioning (to gain and keep patient's attention); when to use targeted questioning patterns (to promote engagement) and when to use humor (to reduce a tense atmosphere). Hopefully, students will equally learn when to listen more than speak (to assist anxious patients to calm down during the history-taking process). In essence, there are also times when it is most appropriate to nod in affirmation as patients speak, when to speak with authority while maintaining eye contact and when to provide narratives of clinical finding during the patient examination process. Subba (2014) posits these styles are implemented with a strategy to help create a tranquil consultation atmosphere, reduce anxiety and fear while promoting the chances for trust development in all settings, including the healthcare settings.

This book will be an excellent resource that can introduce students to the simple steps that can be appropriately implemented through the strategic use of communication styles which will help improve the chances of not only establishing better connections with patients but also reducing the risks of frustrations and burnout in their future healthcare practices.

Nonye Tochi Aghanya, MSc, RN, FNP-C

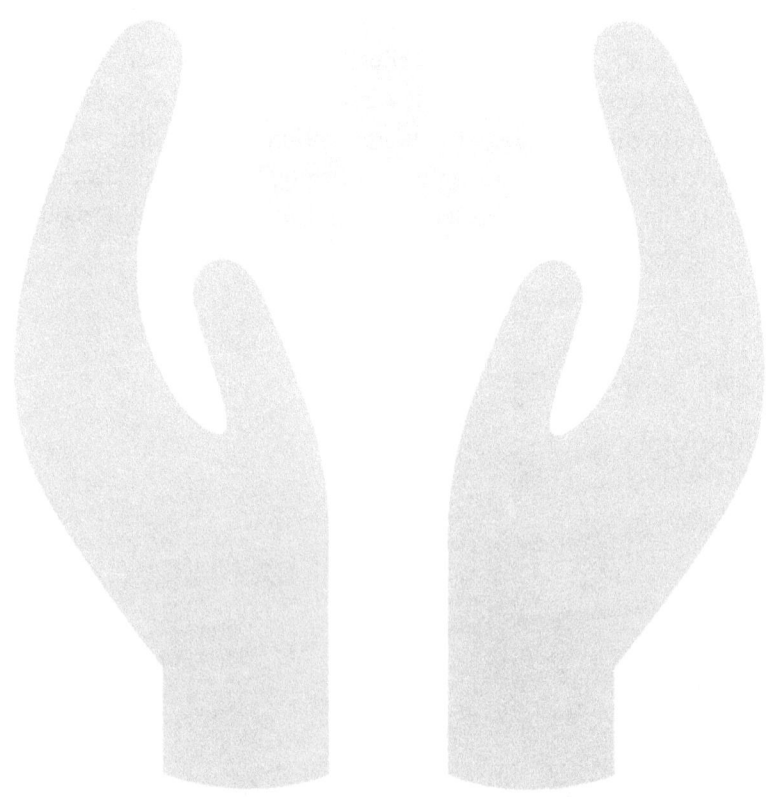

REFERENCES

Aghanya, Nonye T. 2016. *"Simple Tips to Developing a Productive Clinician-Patient Relationship"* IUniverse Publishing.

Aghanya, Nonye T. 2017. *"This Patient Did Not Want My Care Because of How I Looked."* http://bit.ly/2yYTm6Q

Aghanya, Nonye T. 2019. *"Principles for Overcoming Communication, Anxiety and Improving Trust."* Folio Avenue Publishing.

Alexander, Stewart C., Mary E. Cox, C. L. Boling Turner, Pauline Lyna, Truls Ostbye, James A. Tulsky, Rowena J. Dolor, and Kathryn I. Pollak. 2011. "Do the five A's work when Physician's Counsel About Weight Loss?" *Family Medicine* 43(3): 179-84.

https://www.ncbi.nlm.nih.gov/pmc/articles/PMC3367376/

Armstrong, M. J., T.A. Mottershead, P.E Ronksley, R.J. Sigal, T.S. Campbell, and B.R. Hemmelgan. 2011. "Motivational Interviewing to Improve weight loss in overweight and/or obese patients: A systematic review and meta-analysis and randomized controlled trials." *Obesity Reviews* 12(9): 709-23. doi: 10.1111/j.1467-789X.2011.00829.x.

review and meta-analysis and randomized controlled trials." *Obesity Reviews* 12(9): 709-23. doi: 10.1111/j.1467-789X.2011.00829.x.

Banich, Marie T., Kristen Mackiewicz, Brendan E. Depue, Anson Whitmer, Gregory A. Miller, and Wendy Heller. 2009. "Cognitive Control Mechanism, Emotion and Memory: A Neural Perspective with Implications for Psychopathology." *Neuroscience and Behavioral Reviews* 33(5): 613-30. doi: 10.1016/j.neubiorev.2008.09.010.
Brown, Ernest. 2016. "How to Avoid a Sore Arm from a flu shot". Accessed April 3, 2016.

Center for Medicare and Medicaid Services (CMS) and Agency for Healthcare Research and Quality (AHRQ), 2008). "Survey of Patient Experiences". Accessed December 12, 2015. http://www.medicare.gov/hospitalcompare

Choudhry, Asad J., Yaser M. Baghdadi, Amy E. Wagie, Elizabeth B. Habermann, Stephanie F. Heller, Donald H. Jenkins, Daniel C. Cullinane, and Martin D. Zielinski. 2015. "Readability of Discharge Summaries: With what level of Information are we dismissing our patients?" *The American Journal of Surgery* 211(3): 631-36. http://dx.doi.org/10.1016/j.amjsurg.2015.12.005

Empathy decline and its reasons: a systematic review of studies with medical students and residents. Retrieved from https://www.ncbi.nlm.nih.gov/pubmed/21670661

Fiore, Marrecca, Maurie Markman, Michael W. Smith, et al. 2015. "Precision Medicine, Patient Engagement: Your Questions Answered." *Medscape: Perspectives*. Accessed January 2016.

https://www.medscape.com/viewarticle/854732

Fisher, Michael R. 2015. "Educating ourselves: A Lovist or Fearist perspective?" Technical paper no. 54.

"Figure 1 Inc." 296 Richmond Street West, Toronto, Ontario, Canada. M5V 1X2. Accessed January 8, 2015. https://figure1.com/.

Harding, Anne. 2014. "Americans' Trust in Doctors Is Falling". *Livescience*. Accessed March 20, 2016. www.livescience.com/48407-americans-trust-doctors-falling.html

Interactional skills training in undergraduate medical education: Ten principles for guiding future research. Retrieved from https://www.ncbi.nlm.nih.gov/pubmed/31092235

Kalu, Osinakachi A. 2018. "The first stage of the fearologist." CreateSpace Independent Publishing.

Kessler, David. "Because Love Never Dies. The 5 Stages of Grief." Accessed April 2016. http://grief.com/the-five-stages-of-grief.

Krebs, Paul, and Dustin T. Duncan. 2015. "Health App Use Among U.S. Mobile Phone Owners: A National Survey." *JMIR Mhealth and Uhealth* 3(4): e101. doi:10.2196/mhealth.4924

Kushner, Robert F., Caroline M. Apovian, and Donna H. Ryan. 2015. "Obesity Management: Improving Outcomes by Engaging Patients." *Medscape Education Family Medicine*. Accessed November 20, 2015. http://www.medscape.org/viewarticle/851776

Merriam-Webster Collegiate Dictionary. 11th Edition. 2003. Springfield, MA: Merriam-Webster. http://www.merriam-webster.com.

Parkin, Tracey, and Timothy C. Skinner. 2003. "Discrepancies between patients and Professionals recall and Perception of an Outpatient Consultation". *Diabetic Medicine* 20(11): 909-14. Accessed April 10, 2016. doi:10.1046/j.1464-5491.2003.01056.x

Pollak, Kathryn L., Stewart C. Alexander, Cynthia J. Coffman, James A. Tulsky, Pauline Lyna, Rowena J. Dolor, Iguehi E. James, Rebecca J. Namenek Brouwer, Justin R. E. Manusov, and Truls Ostbye. 2010. "Physician Communication Techniques and Weight Loss in Adults: Project CHAT." *American Journal of Preventive Medicine* 39(4): 321-28. doi:10.1016/j.amepre.2010.06.005

Sheppard, Elena. "19 of Maya Angelou's Most Powerful Quotes to Remember Her By." Mic. May 28 2014. Accessed February 12, 2015.
Snyder, Lois. 2012. "American College of Physician Ethics Manual, Sixth Edition." *Annal Internal Medicine* 156: 73-104. doi: 10.7326/0003-4819-156-1-201201031-00001.

Snyder, Lois S., and Jon C Tilburt. 2016. "Maintaining Medical Professionalism Online: Posting of patient Information: A case Study." *American College of Physician Ethics Case Studies*. www.medscape.org/viewarticle/857101

Spring, B., K. Schneider, H.G. McFadden, J. Vaughn, A.T. Kozak, M. Smith, A. C. Moller, L. H. Epstein, A. DeMott, D. Hedeker, J. Siddique, and D. M. Llyod-Jones. 2012. "Multiple Behavior Change in Diet and Activity: A Randomized Controlled Trial Using Mobile Technology." *Archives of Internal Medicine* 172(10): 789-96. doi:10.1001/archinternmed.2012.1044

Subba, D. 2014. "Philosophy of fearism: Life is conducted, directed and controlled by the Fear." XLIBRIS

Teaching empathy to medical students: an updated, systematic review. Retrieved from https://www.ncbi.nlm.nih.gov/pubmed/23807099

Thakkar Jay, Rahul Kurup, Tracey-Lee Laba, Karla Santo, Aravinda Thiagalingam, Anthony Rodgers, Mark Woodward, Julie Redfern, and Clara K. Chow. 2016. "Mobile Telephone Text Messaging for Medication Adherence in Chronic Disease: A Meta-analysis." *JAMA Intern Med* 176(3): 340-49. doi:10.1001/jamainternmed.2015.7667.

Tracey, P. & Skinner, T.C. (2003). Discrepancies between patients and professionals: Recall and perception of an outpatient consultation. Diabetic Medicine, 20(11): 909-14, doi:10.1046/j.1464-5491.2003.01056.x

Trzeciak, S. (2019) . "Is there a Healthcare compassion crisis?" TEDxPenn talk by Dr. Stephen Trzeciak https://bit.ly/2Zy25a2

Trzeciak, S, & Mazzarelli, A. (2019). Compassionomics book: The revolutionary scientific evidence that caring makes a difference. Studer Group

US public health service syphilis study at Tuskegee. Retrieved from https://www.cdc.gov/tuskegee/timeline.htm

Weber, Michael, Jan Basile, David Kountz, and Nancy H. Miller. 2015. "Strategies to Improve Adherence and Persistence in the Treatment of Hypertension." *Medscape Education Cardiology*. Accessed January 21, 2016.
www.medscape.org/viewarticle/849742

Welch, Gilbert H. 2015. "Less Medicine More Health: Seven Assumptions That Drive Too Much Medical Care, Assumption # 4: It Never Hurts to Get Too Much Information." Beacon Press

Nonye Tochi Aghanya, MSc, RN, FNP-C

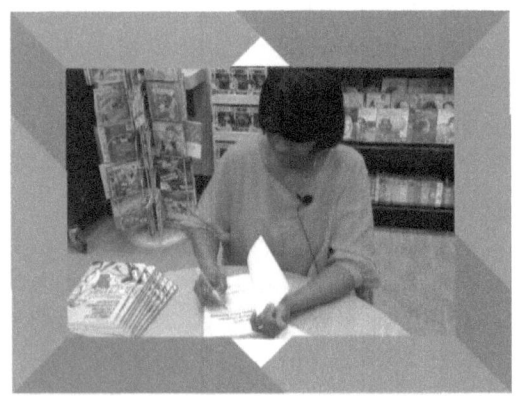

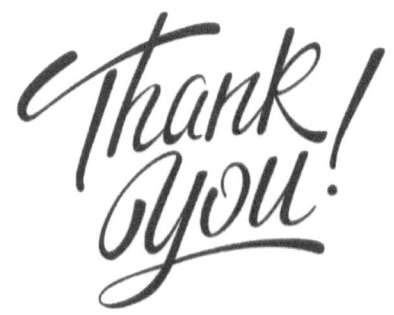

www.ingramcontent.com/pod-product-compliance
Lightning Source LLC
Chambersburg PA
CBHW031414210526
45464CB00005B/1883